Everybody

Derek Llewellyn-Jones wa[...]
lives in Australia, where [...]
Obstetrics and Gynaecolog[...]
1988. He is now a full-tin[...]
Everywoman: A Gynaecolo[...]
Faber, 5th edn., 1990), *The* [...]
2nd edn., 1990), and *Every Man* (OUP, 3rd edn., 1991).

Everybody

The healthy eating handbook

● ●

Derek Llewellyn-Jones

Oxford   Melbourne

OXFORD UNIVERSITY PRESS

1993

Oxford University Press, Walton Street, Oxford OX2 6DP

Oxford New York Toronto
Delhi Bombay Calcutta Madras Karachi
Kuala Lumpur Singapore Hong Kong Tokyo
Nairobi Dar es Salaam Cape Town
Melbourne Auckland Madrid
and associated companies in
Berlin Ibadan

Oxford is a trade mark of Oxford University Press

British Library Cataloguing in Publication Data
Data available

Library of Congress Cataloging in Publication Data
Llewellyn-Jones, Derek.
Everybody: the healthy eating handbook / Derek Llewellyn-Jones.
  p. cm.
Includes index.
1. Nutrition. I. Llewellyn-Jones, Derek. Everybody. II. Title.
RA784.L62 1993   92-19159
ISBN 0–19–286155–7

10 9 8 7 6 5 4 3 2 1

Typeset by Best-set Typesetter Ltd., Hong Kong
Printed in Great Britain by
Clays Ltd.
Bungay, Suffolk

Preface

What you eat, how often you eat, and the substances that are added to the food you eat have a profound effect on your health. You may be surprised to know that in most industrialized countries many people are malnourished—that is, they eat the wrong foods in the wrong proportions. On the other hand, many people in the developing countries are undernourished—that is, they don't have enough to eat. They are also often malnourished.

Until people are aware of the ways in which the right foods promote good health and, conversely, the ways in which the wrong foods can lead to ill health, they are unlikely to change their eating habits.

That is what this book is about. It is about the way in which human beings eat and absorb foodstuffs and liquids. It describes how you use food substances for the production of the energy you need to keep alive, to maintain and repair body tissues, and to ensure that your organs function properly so that you can continue to enjoy good health. It is about the nutritive value of foodstuffs, and the relationships between diet, health, and disease. It is critical of many modern dietary practices and of the way we often encourage ill health by choosing foods that are harmful or have low nutritive benefits. It aims to make you, the reader, think about the foods you eat, and question whether your eating habits are sensible and healthy.

Many books about nutrition and weight reduction contain pages and pages of recipes. You will not find any recipes in *Everybody*. Most readers do not use the recipes in a book like this, or if they do, it isn't for long. It is more important that, after reading this book, you should be able to work out for yourself what to eat for a balanced diet and, if necessary, how to reduce your energy intake.

Contents

List of Figures

1 BODY IMAGE

● ●

We in the West are obsessed by body image. Judging by the number of books published each year, and of articles and advertisements in magazines and newspapers, promoting the ideal of a slim, tanned, and physically fit body, both for men and for women, beauty seems to be big business.

All ideals of beauty, however, are transient: the body features that are considered beautiful in one decade may not necessarily be thought so in the next. At times the shape of the body itself, largely exposed, has been perceived as beautiful and sexually desirable. At other times, fashion has dictated that the body be shrouded in clothes whose design, texture, and shape lend beauty to the body and enhance its sexual attractiveness. The concept of beauty in both sexes, but particularly in women, has fluctuated between conceal-ment and revealment. Manners may make the man, but for much of history, at least after the fourteenth century in Europe, clothes have made the woman. Up to the late four-teenth century, the few rich wore gowns, while the many poor wore tunics or skirts. These clothes concealed the body, rendering it shapeless. But fashion changed, and by the fifteenth century men were wearing clothes that emphasized their genitals, with elaborate codpieces and multicoloured tights. Women continued to wear gowns, but these no longer concealed the body; instead they emphasized the shape of the body and were often cut low to accentuate the breasts.

Such information as we have suggests that in the 500 years since 1500, young women of the wealthier classes have chosen to remain slim, at least until they marry and have children, when some, but by no means all, put on weight. There is less information about the poor, but what there is suggests that most of them were thin.

It is not difficult to see why. Up to 150 years ago there were many years in which food was scarce for the less well off. Food choice was also limited. Until the nineteenth century most people's diet consisted of bread made from barley, wheat, and rye, up to 5 lb. being eaten a day. Soup, a little meat, cheese, vegetables, milk, eggs, and weak ale made up the rest of the diet. For most people, particularly in the rural areas, the morning meal was the main meal. After breaking their nocturnal fast the workers left for the fields, taking with them a snack. On their return late in the evening another meal would be eaten. Clearly few people gave any thought to the shape of their bodies; it was hard enough to keep away hunger.

For the rich the type of food was similar but more plentiful: much more meat and fish were available, although it is doubtful that most of the small number of wealthy people before the eighteenth century ate excessively.

Among the poor, the women were the bearers and rearers of children. They worked in the house and in the fields, and their days were long and arduous. According to a French eighteenth-century writer, peasant women lost any beauty they may have had early in life: 'sunburn, sweat and continual fatigue impair their features and their figure. Before the age of eighteen, girls who elsewhere would have been pleasing and pretty have suntanned skins, horny hands and a stoop.' Only among the rich was a woman expected to be beautiful and idle, gracing her father's and then her husband's house, and her life was arranged to fit in with this conceit.

An agricultural revolution took place in England from the middle of the eighteenth century to the early nineteenth century. Open fields were enclosed into smaller rectangular fields where scientific rotation of crops could be conducted, and stock were fed to become fat. Waste land, old woodland, heath, thickets, and swamps were cleared or drained to make more arable land available. Estates were enlarged and consolidated, and transport by canal, sea, and road made the movement of goods and people quicker and easier. Winter grass and roots were grown and stored so that for the first time cattle and sheep could be fed during the winter, and the wholesale slaughter of stock in the autumn was avoided. Salt meat was replaced by fresh beef and mutton. The improvement of the land led to bigger harvests of wheat, which now grew where oats, barley, and rye had grown before.

These improvements in food supply were countered by a rapid increase in population (which rose from 9 million in 1801 to 20 million in 1851), and a rise in the number of landless labourers. This in turn led to migration to the towns. In 1801 only 17 per cent of the population lived in towns; by 1857 this had risen to 50 per cent. Overall the average person, and in particular those living in the towns, ate no better than previously, and hunger was common.

By the mid nineteenth century the changes in agricultural practice had made a greater variety of foods available, at least for those who could afford it. The middle class and the rich ate well; the poor, living in overcrowded conditions, had more food than before, but adulteration of bread and milk, which made up most of their diet, was common.

By the 1870s corn from America and refrigerated meat from Australia and New Zealand added further to the variety of foods available, but even with this many people went hungry.

It is not surprising that the ideal body shape, which at this time emphasized the breasts of women and the legs of men, was of concern only to the rich and some of the middle class. The ideal woman was one who had a pretty face, full breasts, and a wasp-waist. The mid-Victorians may have appeared inhibited and strait-laced on the outside, but they were as sexually active as people in other more 'permissive' periods. There are numerous pornographic postcards, *cartes de visite*, produced in abundance in France from about 1860, which show naked women with full breasts, buttocks and thighs, and a slightly protuberant belly. There are few pictures of naked men, and such as exist show men of muscular build.

Why there are so few pictures of naked men is not clear. The novelist and art critic John Berger has suggested: '*men act* and *women appear*. Men look at women. Women watch themselves being looked at. This determines not only most relations between men and women but also the relation of women to themselves. The surveyor of woman in herself is male: the surveyed female. Thus she turns herself into an object—and most particularly an object of vision: a sight'. Berger suggests that men may derive their ideal of female beauty from visual images, and that women respond by trying to live up to that ideal.

Since the First World War many more women have been more aware of the shape of their bodies and have taken action to bring it into line with the current fashion. During the war the shortage of labour to make uniforms, and to work in munition and other factories gave women the opportunity to escape their limited, poorly paid drudgery in shops or in service before marriage, and in their own homes after marriage. This change, together with the beginning of women's political emancipation, led to a change in the perception of many women about their body shape. The New Woman was created. The padded, corseted, long-skirted young women became the flappers of the 1920s, who rejected the full-breasted, narrow-waisted concept of feminine beauty of the later Victorian and Edwardian periods, and chose to be slim with small breasts.

Between the wars, the ideal shape of women's bodies continued to change: sometimes full breasts were seen as attractive, at other times small was beautiful; but increasingly fashion dictated that clothes reveal the shape of the body rather than concealing it.

The new body shape could be achieved by many women only if they reduced the amount of food they ate, and exercised. Dieting and exercise began to become fashionable.

The Second World War gave a further impetus to women's 'liberation' and an increased awareness of body shape and image. The perceived desirability of slimness persisted, encouraged by images of women in newspapers and magazines, and then by the most invasive and persuasive of all the media, television.

Studies in the 1950s, 1960s, and 1970s confirm that slimness was seen as desirable by women and appreciated by men. A study of the 'vital statistics' of *Playboy* centrefold models and of competitors in the finals of the Miss America pageant since 1960 shows that although the breast size preferred by the judges has varied and there has been a small increase in the preferred height of the women, the weight of the winners has decreased and is below the average weight of American women of similar age and height. Feminists may argue that this demonstrates the continued oppression of women by men, but it can be argued as strongly that the women themselves feel more comfortable, assured, and confident if they are slim rather than fat.

The message from the media since the Second World War has encouraged the idea that the happiest, most successful years of life are one's youth, and that a woman will be more successful in employment and in relationships if she is slim. For men the emphasis is on having a muscular, sporting figure: wimps and nerds are out. This is why so many gyms, with elaborate body-building apparatus, have appeared in the last twenty years.

In the 1960s studies of American and Swedish teenagers demonstrated that the young women were particularly concerned about their body shape and weight. Fifteen years later, in the 1980s, further comparable studies showed that women's perceptions as to what body shape and weight was desirable had not changed.

In these studies nearly half the women perceived themselves as being heavier than they really were, and one-third considered themselves to be fat, although measurement of their height and weight showed that they were not. Over three-quarters of the teenagers wanted to lose weight, one woman in four was worried about overeating, and one in five was fearful that unless she dieted she would gain too much weight.

Further investigations about women's perception of their

body shape have shown that many women of all ages want to lose weight from particular parts of their body. For example, a study conducted in Australia in 1987 showed that 75 per cent of the women questioned wanted to have smaller thighs, smaller hips, and a smaller 'stomach', while 65 per cent thought that their bottom was too large. Many of the women took measures to lose weight. Between one-third and two-thirds of the women dieted from time to time, and one woman in six dieted 'seriously'. Another method of losing weight was vigorous exercise. Only a few resorted to potentially dangerous methods of weight loss—self-induced vomiting or laxative abuse.

The evidence is that many women, particularly young women, and some men, in most Western countries, are under enormous pessure to be trim, taut, and tanned. Commercial advertising, soap operas on television, and films portray the heroes as slim and muscular, and the heroines as young, beautiful, and usually slim. Fat men and women play comic characters. Women's magazines feature glamorous models who are usually thin. Popular newspapers add to the perception that to 'succeed' a woman should be slim and beautiful, and a man slim and muscular.

To meet the perceived demand, the commercial weight-loss industry is flourishing. Magazine articles and books regularly feature exciting new diets that promise to melt away fat painlessly and quickly. The diets can't work that well, as they are soon replaced by new diets in a new article or a new book.

There is an intense interest in body shape and weight in most developed countries. Everybody is interested in their body, not necessarily for reasons of better health but because a good body shape is equated with better self-esteem and with 'success' in relationships.

2 PHYSICAL ACTIVITY

• •

> It is not the rich and the great, nor those who depend
> on medicine, who become old: but such as use much
> exercise. For the idler never attains great age.
>
> Thomas Easton, 1799

As this book has been written to provide information about
ways in which you can keep your body as healthy and in as
good shape as you would wish, it is appropriate to consider
healthy exercise habits as well as healthy eating habits.

Until the late 1700s most working people in all countries
engaged in a good deal of physical activity in their everyday
lives. Over 85 per cent of the population lived in rural areas
and followed rural pursuits. The seasonal cycle of farming,
the cottage industries, the need to carry water from wells
and to grow and gather food from cottage gardens demanded
a good deal of physical activity. Only the landed gentry and
the shopkeepers in the towns did not have to expend much
physical energy, but the former, at least, exerted themselves
in outdoor sports.

The Industrial Revolution during the next century and a
half changed the pattern of physical activity. Machine power
replaced muscle power to a large extent, although human
labour was still required.

By the mid twentieth century, when fewer than 20 per cent
of people in developed countries lived in rural areas, most
workers, even in jobs involving heavy machinery, did not
need to expend much muscle power. The increasingly sophisticated machines took care of most of the energy needs.
Although physical labour was still employed in farming,
many of the tasks previously done by people were now done

by machines. Cottage industries had almost completely disappeared, and women who had manufactured goods on a small, labour-intensive scale were now joining the work-force in factories and offices, where monotonous, repetitive actions were required which demanded little muscle power. Buses, trains, and cars replaced feet as a means of getting to the work-place and the shops. Television, watched by each person for an average of twelve hours a week, filled much leisure time.

It is not surprising that over half of men, and nearly two-thirds of women, in several developed countries rarely or never engage in recreational physical activity, and very few engage in recreational physical activity three times a week.

There is, of course, a minority of men and women who play strenuous games, jog or walk for pleasure, go to gyms, participate in aerobic exercises, or enjoy body-building. This group is getting bigger, as evidenced by the growing number of gyms, and of books, often written by or ghost-written for media personalities, that suggest that if you follow the regimen of exercise promoted you can become fit and healthy: if you are male you can become more muscular and macho; if you are female you can become more trim and beautiful.

Is there any benefit in taking regular physical activity? If there is, as Thomas Easton suggested 200 years ago, why don't more people become healthier by taking regular exercise?

The majority of people are slothful, and although some say that they would engage in regular exercise if they could, they find reasons for not doing so. In 1985 the Australian Better Health Commission enquired about the physical activity of over 1,000 randomly selected Australians. They were asked whether they thought their future health could be improved if they changed their life-style. Three-quarters of those interviewed thought that their health would be improved if they made changes. One-quarter selected increased exercise as the most useful change that they could make. However, when asked why they had not made the change to take more exercise, they gave two main reasons. The first, subscribed to by 47 per cent of the respondents, was that they 'had no time'. The second, given by 32 per cent of the respondents, was that they were too lazy.

The benefits of frequent, regular physical exertion have been investigated and reported on. One major benefit is in improving the function of the cardiovascular system, which reduces the risk of a heart attack, and may reduce the level of blood pressure. Another benefit of exercise is that, combined with a programme of reduced intake of energy from food, it enables an overweight or obese person to lose weight more quickly and to maintain the lower weight. A third benefit is that it keeps the muscles strong and the joints supple. Strength and suppleness make many everyday tasks easier to perform and help to prevent aches and pains and the development of arthritis. Yet another benefit of regular exercise that is perceived by the person as enjoyable is that it promotes a feeling of well-being. This may be due to the release of certain hormones (endorphins) during exercise which produce a 'high'; or it may be because during exercise one can escape from one's worries.

There are two main kinds of physical exertion. The first is designed to improve the performance of the heart and the respiratory system. This is achieved by aerobic exercises. Aerobic exercises promote the ability of the body to use oxygen more efficiently. They include any type of exercise that uses large muscle groups, makes the heart work harder, and causes one to become slightly breathless. To benefit the cardiovascular and respiratory systems, the aerobic exercises must make the heart work above a certain threshold, and the exercises need to be repeated about three times a week for thirty minutes. A handy guide is for you to engage in aerobic exercises that increase your heart rate to 190 beats per minute minus your age.

Aerobic physical activity can be graded. Vigorous exercise includes playing squash or running 3 k in fifteen minutes. Moderate aerobic physical activity includes walking briskly for thirty minutes, jogging 2 k in fifteen minutes, or swimming. You should do one of these three times a week.

If you embark on a fitness programme using an aerobic exercise, you may expect to obtain some protection against a heart attack, because the physical activity trains the heart to do less work to meet the demands made on it. Aerobic exercise also speeds the blood flow through the arteries and alters the blood lipids in a favourable direction, so that atheromas are prevented or perhaps reduced in size.

The physical activity has to be engaged in regularly, as the benefits are reversed in about six weeks if the exercises are abandoned and you become slothful again. Nearly half of all people joining aerobic exercise classes give up within a year.

Exercises to improve muscle strength and joint flexibility are contained in many aerobic programmes, but if you are interested only in body-building so as to feel more attractive, isometric exercises, in which you strain your muscle groups against resistance, will meet that need. However, isometric exercises offer no protection against heart disease. In fact, if you have heart disease, you should avoid isometric exercises.

The choice of an exercise programme depends on what you

....

Principles of Enjoyable Physical Exercise

- The exercise chosen should be perceived as enjoyable.
- The programme should be graded, and gradually increased.
- The exercise programme should be engaged in regularly, usually three times a week, for twenty to thirty minutes depending on the exercise chosen.
- The programme should not produce severe discomfort. The concept that 'there is no gain without pain' should be rejected. It is foolish!
- In most cases the exercises should start with a warm-up period and end with a cool-down period. During these times gentle stretching of muscle groups should be undertaken to reduce the chance of injury.
- Strenuous exercise should not be engaged in soon after a large meal, or in conditions of high heat and humidity. Drink plenty of water.

....

are looking for. The main criterion should be that you see the exercise programme as enjoyable and are thus motivated to persist with it. Some people enjoy playing squash or tennis; some enjoy jogging; some prefer brisk walking; some choose to go to aerobic exercise classes. The choice should be the individual's.

The finding that fewer than half the adults in most developed countries engage in regular physical activity suggests that a change in behaviour is required if the health benefits of exercise on the body and mind are to be achieved. There is no obvious solution, given the competing attractions of television, the pub, and attending (rather than participating in) sporting events.

One suggestion is that a convenient time for people to learn new habits is during the school years. Studies of schools where physical-fitness programmes have been introduced show that there have been health benefits. Studies in Australia and Canada show that in a comparison of the 'fitness group' (who engaged in three to five hours of fairly vigorous physical activity a week) and the 'standard group' (who did the traditional Physical Education (PE) programme), the skills and behaviour of the students in the fitness group were superior to that of the control group.

A problem with these studies is that the programme was carried out for only a short period, and there was no guarantee that the students would continue with it in their leisure hours or after leaving school.

Of course many teenagers and young adults take part in sport, and this is to be encouraged, but no assessment has been made as to whether these people have fewer heart attacks and more mobile joints in later life. Because so many life-style changes take place over the years, it is impossible to determine if a correlation between the two exists. The athlete of today may become a couch-potato in the next decade. But if people continue to take regular enjoyable exercise three times a week, the chances are that they will be healthier and physically more fit as they grow into middle age.

3 DIETARY CRAZES AND CRAZY DIETS

● ●

It is a sad paradox that, with the increasing availability of education and a wider range of information, people still persist in believing in magical remedies to avoid, or to cure, many diseases of modern civilization. Many people remain convinced that a copper bangle worn on the wrist will alleviate rheumatism; thousands, in desperation, seek worthless 'cancer cures', often at incapacitating expense. Similarly, millions consume large quantities of unnecessary vitamin and mineral supplements every day, which pass through their bodies unchanged, only to enrich the sewage.

In no area of health do magical remedies play a greater part than in the control of obesity. As a society we are hooked on crazy diets and have a succession of dietary crazes. In 1989 a survey of a number of women's magazines in the USA, Britain, and Australia showed that on average a new diet, which claimed to be highly effective, was published in every third issue, only to be superseded by a diet which claimed to be even more effective in the next issue but two. The desire of people in affluent countries to lose weight quickly, painlessly, and with as little disturbance to their way of life as possible is the basis for the proliferation of diets. Faith persuades them that the new diet will enable them to achieve this objective.

The modern obsession with dieting is also very profitable. Books about diet, if well publicized and promoted, sell millions of copies, especially in the USA. Food fads and cults attract millions of people, who part with their money for the dubious, and usually temporary, satisfaction of 'feeling better'.

Food provides energy, and in an isolated system—such as a human being—energy follows the first law of thermodynamics: 'The energy in an isolated system is constant: any exchange of energy between a system and its surroundings must occur with the creation or destruction of energy.' If more energy is absorbed than is lost, weight gain is inevitable.

As people enjoy eating and want to lose weight without having to avoid the foods they like (which are usually high in energy), diets were published from the late 1940s which, the authors claimed, would permit people to eat most of the foods they liked and still lose weight. These diets had two common features. First, the dieters did not have to restrict their total energy intake: they could eat as much protein and fat as they liked. Second, they had to eat few or no carbohydrates (both simple and complex carbohydrates).

The first diet in this century that confidently said you could eat fat and get thin was introduced by Dr Alfred Pennington in 1953. He believed that fat people were fat because their metabolism quickly turned almost all the carbohydrate they ate into fat. He argued from this that if you cut out carbohydrate almost completely, you could eat as much fat and protein as you liked and you would lose weight. But you should eat fat and protein in a ratio of 1 to 3. In other words, you had to eat fat meat.

About eight years later, in 1961, the 'Pennington principle' was elaborated on by Dr Herman Taller in a book called *Calories don't Count*. He believed that by eating lots of 'the right fats' (mainly polyunsaturated fats) you set in motion a process which burned up not only the fat you ate but also all the fats you had accumulated over the years in your adipose tissue.

Several other diets followed which ignored the first law of thermodynamics. It did not seem to matter. Satisfied clients provided 'proof' that the diets worked, perhaps because dissatisfied clients did not bother to tell anyone. Dieting had become big business.

One of most popular books, judging by sales, was Dr Stillman's *The Doctor's Quick Weight Loss Diet*. Dr Stillman agreed that calories did not need to be limited and that carbohydrates needed to be nearly eliminated, but he discouraged the dieter from eating fats. He said that the diet should be rich in protein, which he claimed would in some mysterious way melt away fat stores. In addition, the dieter had to drink at least eight glasses of water each day, presumably to 'flush the kidneys'. For seven years Dr Stillman's diet found a ready market and was used, for a short time, by thousands of overweight Americans. Then in 1974 its effectiveness or lack of effectiveness was investigated by a team of medical scientists. They found that although people on the diet were allowed to eat as much protein as they wished, their protein intake increased only to 160 g a day compared with an average American man's intake of 100 g. At the same time their fat intake fell below that eaten by an average American, from 115 g to 73 g a day. As the dieters were severely restricting their carbohydrate intake, and in consequence their fat intake ('if you don't eat bread how do you eat butter'), their total energy intake fell by nearly half. And of course the dieter lost weight, mostly during the first four weeks of the diet, but not at the rate of 5 to 15 lb. claimed by Dr Stillman. Scientists found that, unfortunately for the dieter, the loss was transient, being due to the severe restriction of carbohydrate, particularly complex carbohydrate, which led to a loss of glycogen and water from the glycogen–water pool. They also found that many of the dieters complained of fatigue, mild nausea, or diarrhoea, and most could not adhere to the diet for longer than six weeks. They concluded: 'There seems very little reason for recommending the Stillman diet.' This opinion was then put more forcibly by the spokesman for the American Medical Association's Council on Foods and Nutrition, Dr Phillip White, who wrote: 'It is essentially planned malnutrition. If you followed the diet as directed, you would actually lose protein from vital organs and other parts of the body. These losses could be quite devastating to somebody in poor health.'

In 1972 Dr Atkins, a fashionable New York physician, published his 'revolutionary diet', which was syndicated in women's magazines, and then published as a hardback book carrying an evangelical dedication: 'to all diet revolutionaries who are not content merely to follow their own diet but who are dedicated to carrying the message of the diet revolution to the world that needs it'. These were stirring words but not true.

The diet in the book was neither as new nor as revolutionary as Dr Atkins claimed. Once again it was a low-carbohydrate, high-fat, moderate-protein diet. It was written in easily digestible sections, interspersed with anecdotes of the diet's success among the rich, the famous, and the notorious. 'Imagine losing weight with a diet that lets you have bacon and eggs for breakfast, heavy cream in your coffee, plenty of meat, and even salad *with* dressing for lunch and dinner', said the blurb. The appeal to the affluent and overfed, who craved the good things of life but wanted to lose weight, met with instant success. Millions of copies of the book were sold.

One of the ways in which the diet was supposed to melt weight from the body was that it produced ketones. Ketones are produced when fat is burned to provide energy when there is insufficient carbohydrate in the diet and the glycogen–water pool has been exhausted. Dr Atkins claimed that the ketones 'sneaked hundreds of calories out of your body every day' in some unexplained way. Unfortunately ketones do not, as two medical scientists reported after evaluating the diet. They concluded that the maximum loss of calories due to the ketones in the diet was 50 kcal a day, far fewer than the 'hundreds of calories' promised.

The successor to Dr Atkins's diet was the Scarsdale Medical Diet, which appeared in 1978 and is still in print. The diet was a low-carbohydrate and low-fat diet, which was monotonous and nutritionally unbalanced. The first fourteen days of the diet, during which the person was 'guaranteed' to lose 20 lb. was strict: very little food was eaten. In addition, the diet limited the amount of fluid (only tea and coffee) that might be drunk. During this time most of the weight lost was water. After two weeks the dieter was permitted to eat more, as long as he or she kept to the monotonous fixed menu. The diet was analysed by nutritionists and found to be dangerous to health.

All these diets were nutritionally unsound, as they contained very small quantities of complex carbohydrates. They were also psychologically unsound, as they were rather unpalatable, which led to most dieters abandoning them before long to return to a more palatable diet. Although a considerable loss of weight occurred in the first two or three weeks of the diets (due mainly to a loss of water), the dieter's weight tended to increase rapidly after the initial loss as the dehydration was reversed, and then a small weight loss occurred each week. But the monotony of the diet demanded a high degree of motivation to persevere and persist with it. Most people did not have it.

Another approach to health through diet and weight reduction emerged in the late 1960s, in the days of flower power and Zen. These were the Zen Macrobiotic Diets, which, it was claimed, worked wonders. The diets consisted of several 'levels' through which the dieter assiduously worked. The Zen diets have been condemned by nutritionists as potentially dangerous, as they have led, in some people, to damaged kidney function, anaemia, and emaciation. Emaciation may be all right for meditation, but it is not a healthy state.

In the late 1970s a new guru of dieting appeared, whose diet did not eliminate complex carbohydrates and in fact encouraged the person to eat more of them. The diet also had the advantage that it was nutritionally sound. Nathan Pritikin, who had heart disease, developed a diet—the Pritikin Diet—which he claimed was 'the world's healthiest diet'. The diet was a restricted diet, in which the dieter was forbidden to eat any fat or refined carbohydrate. It excluded all dairy products, though a little skimmed milk was allowed. Lean meat or fish was not allowed, except in some circumstances, where up to 0.5 kg (1½ lb.) a week was permitted. Complex carbohydrates were eaten to provide up to 80 per

cent of the daily energy intake, but only if they were unprocessed (rye flakes, rolled oats, cracked wheat, raw bran)
or wholegrain. The diet did not permit white bread, white
rice, or pasta. The dieter could eat vegetables (with a few
exceptions) in any quantity, but these were to be eaten raw
or lightly steamed. Fresh fruit was limited. Salt and salty
foods were forbidden.

The Pritikin diet is a nutritious diet, so it cannot be classi-
fied as a crazy diet, but it includes restrictions and prohibi-
tions that diminish its scientific value. Moreover, it does
not meet the criteria for a diet to which a less than highly
motivated person would adhere. (These criteria are discussed
on page 156.)

In the early 1970s liquid diets had appeared, particularly in
the USA. A popular one was the Swedish Liquid Diet, and
several almost identical diets were published with different
names. The idea behind these diets was that the dieter ate no
food and drank only a semi-synthetic mixture of substances
such as dried skimmed milk or soya bean powder, which
provided protein, with a trace of sugar, a dollop of vitamins,
and a slurp of minerals. The total energy content of the diet
was less than 3,200 kJ (800 kcal). New versions of the Swedish
Liquid Diet subsequently appeared which provided even less
energy (1,250–1,800 kJ or 300–430 kcal) a day. These diets are
the Cambridge Diet, the Very Low Calorie Diet, and the
Liquid Protein Diet. They are also available as commercial
products. In the first week of the diet the person loses more
than 5 kg, but after that the weight loss is usually less than
1.5 kg a week. The loss is not only of adipose tissue, but also
of muscle tissue, including heart muscle, the heart becoming
smaller, which means that protein is lost as well as fat.

These diets can pose dangers to one's health and should
not be started unless one is under *direct* medical supervision
and then only after conventional weight-losing programmes
have failed. Without medical supervision, death may occur,
as happened in the USA in the late 1970s when sixty healthy
Americans with no history of heart disease died from heart
failure while on the diet. Moreover, liquid diets break one of

the principles of a good weight-reducing diet, that the diet should be sufficiently palatable and varied to prevent the dieter becoming bored with it quickly. Most dieters trying this diet give up within four to eight weeks. The diet is discussed further on page 29.

In the late 1970s a new popular gimmick appeared. This was the suggestion that a diet composed of a single food, such as eggs or fruit, taken in a strict sequence would have the effect of reducing weight without side-effects. It was an attractive concept for overweight people. It was claimed that if you chose the diet you could continue eating your favourite foods and still lose weight. The diets included the Drinking Man's Diet, the Spaghetti Diet, the Milk and Banana Diet, and many others. The Hard-Boiled Egg Diet was one of these. Hard-boiled eggs, but not soft-boiled eggs or raw eggs, it was claimed, were able, in some mysterious way, to use more energy as they were digested than they released in the body. The diet was rubbish, of course.

More appealing were the fruit diets, as fruit is perceived to be healthy. One of these diets was the Grapefruit Diet, which consisted of nothing more than grapefruit supplemented by a small quantity of bacon and eggs. The grapefruit juice was supposed to dissolve fat, in some miraculous way. In some of the Grapefruit Diets published, it was claimed that you could eat as much bacon and as many eggs as you wished, provided you ate enough grapefruit. There is no scientific merit in the Grapefruit Diet or in similar fruit diets. They do not work. Grapefruit juice has no fat-dissolving powers, but the acidity of the juice might so disturb the person's taste-buds that the craving for sweet foods would be reduced for a time, thus giving the appearance of success.

The fruit diets culminated in the Beverly Hills Diet, whose name obviously capitalized on the glamour and fashion-ableness of Hollywood. The diet consisted of the consump-tion of nothing but certain designated fruits (notably exotic fruits such as mango and papaya), eaten in a specific order, for ten days, after which some bread, meat, and salads could be added. The theory behind this diet is unscientific, and in

1981 the diet was severely criticized by the American Medical Association as nutritionally unsound and dangerous.

In the 1980s fibre became important to health, as is described in Chapter 8. This led to a number of books that promoted dietary fibre as the way to avoid many illnesses. One of the most popular was Audrey Eyton's *The F-Plan Diet*. While the concept of the need for additional dietary fibre in most Western diets was sound, some of the opinions advanced in the books were suspect.

In the late 1980s the dangers of high blood cholesterol re-emerged after some fifteen years' obscurity. Again, authors were not slow to write books promoting diets that claimed to reduce a person's blood cholesterol quickly, painlessly, and without much alteration to dietary habits. The most popular in terms of sales was Robert Kowolsky's *The 8 Week Cholesterol Cure*. The diet worked for some people for a time and their cholesterol level dropped, but over a longer period the diet failed to live up to its promise.

Frequent attempts at new (and scientifically suspect) diets may have further disadvantages. There is evidence that 'weight cycling' or 'yo-yo dieting', in other words losing weight quickly and gaining it again quickly, progressively increases the body's resistance to weight loss, while making weight gain easier. There is now also a belief that 'weight cycling' may increase a person's risk of developing diabetes, high blood pressure, and coronary heart disease.

In addition to the books promoting this or that diet to improve health or reduce weight, during the last fifty years books have appeared regularly which advise their readers about nutrition and how to avoid illness by diet. Many of these books stressed the need for vitamin and mineral supplements. Three of them have endured. Two are by Adelle Davis, who died in 1975, and are entitled *Let's Eat Right to Keep Fit* and *Let's Get Well*. The third is by her successor, Charlton Fredericks, called *Food Facts and Fallacies*.

The books offered some good nutritional advice, particularly at a time when the diet of many Americans was high in fat and sugar, but they contained a large number of errors, some potentially dangerous to health. Dr George Mann, a nutritionist, examined *Let's Eat Right to Keep Fit* and found on average one nutritional or medical error on every page. Professor Rynearson, Emeritus Professor of Medicine at the Mayo Clinic, examined *Let's Get Well* and found a large number of claims that were deceptive and potentially dangerous. Some of Adelle Davis's deceptive claims, for example, were that niacin (one of the B vitamins) prevented 'blue Mondays'; that inositol (another possible B vitamin) cured baldness; and that calcium was a good pain-killer. The potentially dangerous claims were more serious. She suggested that vitamin A should be taken in large doses for a long period to improve health (in fact, it may cause liver damage), that vitamin E cured muscular dystrophy, and that pregnant women should not drink skimmed milk 'because it might cause cataracts in the baby'. The claims were not only false, but could cause much distress.

Charlton Fredericks's book *Food Facts and Fallacies* is aptly described by its title. It is a mixture of facts, fallacies, and fantasies about food and nutrition, but it does contain some good nutritional advice. He recommended that Americans should use less sugar and drink fewer sugar-laden drinks, and that 'a reducing diet should be a miniature of a normal diet, so framed that expansion of the size of the portions will permit the diet to be used *after* weight loss has been stopped'. He condemned the use of hormones, starvation diets, and drugs in the treatment of obesity. These nuggets of good nutritional advice are embedded in a matrix of medical and nutritional misinformation and speculation.

In defence of these authors, it must be said that they were skilled communicators and were critical of many people's food choices and habits at a time when most of the medical profession was silent on such matters. For example, Adelle Davis attacked the habit of giving babies glucose water before lactation was established, and promoted breast-feeding at a time when many doctors made little effort to change infant feeding practices. Adelle Davis's books are still in print; some of the glaring errors have been removed, but a good deal of misinformation remains.

There continues to be a demand for books on food and nutrition. Each year new books appear which give nutritional advice to groups of the population. Many have an almost religious fervour: if you accept their good news you will be healthier, happier, and live longer. They can't really work, or there would not be a market for new books.

It is clear that people continue to be greatly interested in books and magazine articles that claim to help them achieve glowing health or a trim figure or both, without much change in their life-style or in the food they eat. As Professor J. S. Garrow wrote about obesity in 1974: 'Any literate person in a developed country has access to virtually unlimited advice on how to lose weight and much of this advice is misleading . . . There is probably no other field of medicine in which commercial pressures operate so directly against rational treatment.'

4 FAT PEOPLE ARE FAT BECAUSE...

•••••••••••••••••••••••••••••••

To understand why some people become fat it helps to know a little about energy intake and energy expenditure. To remain alive, your body needs energy to power the unconscious functions of breathing, heartbeat, heat control, digestion, and excretion; to replace worn-out tissues with new tissues; and to meet all the other unconscious activities that make up your resting metabolic rate (RMR).

Every time you make a conscious decision to use a group of muscles, to change your position when sitting, to walk around the house, or to undertake physical exertion you need additional energy. If your energy intake is less than your energy expenditure, you have to obtain the extra energy you need from one of two sources. (The exception is when you are very ill, when you may be given the energy you need by an intravenous infusion of nutrients. This is called total parenteral feeding.) The first of these sources is the glycogen–water pool, and the second is the fat stored in your adipose (or fatty) tissue.

The glycogen–water pool has been given this name, although it is not really a pool, because energy in the form of glycogen is stored between the muscle fibres, together with a considerable amount of water. The glycogen–water pool weighs about 4 kg, of which 1 kg is glycogen and the rest water. When glycogen is metabolized it releases 17 kJ (4 kcal) of energy for each gram of glycogen burned. This means that the energy held in the glycogen–water pool will provide about 17,000 kJ or 4,000 kcal, should it be needed, before becoming exhausted. But for every gram of glycogen burned, 3 g of water is lost to the body.

The fat in your adipose tissue is the major source of stored energy, and every gram of adipose tissue burned makes available about 25 kJ or 6 kcal of energy to the body.

If, on the other hand, you absorb more energy from food than you expend in your unconscious and conscious activities, the surplus energy is stored in your body, nearly all of it in adipose tissue as fat, and you put on weight.

Take the amount of energy absorbed by your body from food and subtract from it the amount of energy used for your resting metabolic rate and the energy used in conscious muscle activity, and you have obtained your energy balance.

This can be stated as:

Energy balance = energy intake − energy expenditure

The longer you continue to take in more energy than you expend, the more likely you are to become overweight or obese.

In affluent societies in the West, where over a quarter of adults are overweight or obese, obesity is considered by many physicians to be a major health hazard. In our society most of us can afford, and obtain, a surfeit of rich food and drink: every day can be a feast day. Most of us can guard against heat loss by wearing warm clothes and living in warm houses. Most of us need to take minimal exercise to complete our daily tasks. For these reasons most of us eat more food than we need, that is we take in more energy than we use. The extra energy is converted into fat and stored in our adipose tissue. As the amount of adipose tissue increases we become overweight. Some of us become obese.

The degree to which obesity is a health hazard is debatable. Dr George Mann, an American nutritionist, claims that only gross obesity carries health hazards. He is concerned that too many experts view obesity as a moral issue and write about it in a moralistic manner. The resultant guilt

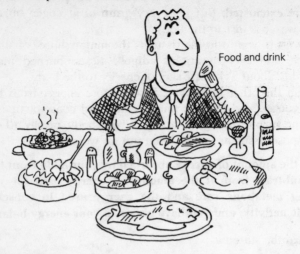

FIG. 4.1. *Energy intake*

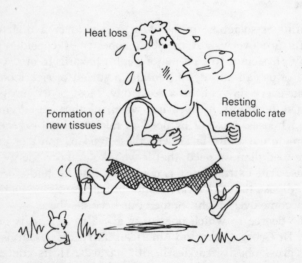

FIG. 4.2. *Energy expenditure*

induced in fat people drives many of them into the hands of quacks—medically qualified and unqualified—or con-men. The quacks wax rich (and often fat!), while their 'patients' all too often remain fat and guilty. Crazy diets, food fads, and dietary crazes cost the British public over £40 million and the American public over $900 million a year.

In poor, hungry societies, fatness is a sign of wealth and a protection against an unexpected famine. In our society, famine is unlikely and a protective layer of fat is unnecessary. However, according to Dr Mann, fatness has certain other uses—flotation, insulation, and flirtation. But since few of us spend much time in water, and most of us can insulate ourselves in cold weather with clothes and central heating, flirtation seems to be the only practical advantage of obesity!

Dr Mann is correct in one way. The experience of many doctors who treat obesity is that the more obese a person is, the more difficult he or she finds it to keep to a weight-reducing diet. The decision to lose weight must, in general, be a personal choice, unless the obesity is so gross that it affects the heart or joints, or aggravates an existing disease, such as diabetes. In these cases the doctor may insist that an overweight patient loses weight. The problem is when such a person often refuses to take advice and appears unconcerned about the effects of gross obesity. But an even greater problem is that people who are only slightly overweight become unduly concerned and depressed about their weight.

Perhaps the best approach is this: if you are overweight and want to reduce your weight so that it lies within the normal range for your height, sex, physique, and age, and if you are prepared to accept the self-discipline of a weight-reducing programme, then go ahead. But if you feel the ordeal would be too great, just carry on eating.

Dr Mann's defence of moderate obesity is opposed by most physicians who have observed that obesity seems to contribute to ill health. This is considered later in the chapter.

There are several ways of determining if you are obese and the severity of your obesity. A convenient way is to weigh yourself and to record your weight in kilograms. Then measure your height and record it in metres. You can now make a calculation to determine your body mass index (BMI), which is:

$$\frac{\text{weight in kilograms}}{\text{height in metres} \times \text{height in metres}}$$

The normal ranges of the body mass index are:

	Men	Women
Underweight	under 20	under 19
Normal weight	20.0–24.9	19.0–24.9
Overweight	25.0–29.9	25.0–29.9
Obese	30 and over	30 and over

You can check your BMI by doing the calculation or by referring to Figure 13.1 (page 154).

In most Western developed countries obesity is fairly common. In Britain, as an example of a developed country, one person in ten over the age of 20 is obese. As a person grows older, obesity is more likely to occur, and the prevalence of obesity peaks between the ages of 55 and 65, when about 18 per cent of women and 14 per cent of men are obese (Figure 4.3)

The BMI is a helpful measure of obesity, but you may want to know how much fat you have in your body. A simple way of doing this is to measure your skin-folds: grasp the skin and underlying tissues over your lower rib-cage between your finger and thumb. If the skin-fold between your finger and thumb is more than 2.5 cm (1 in.) thick, you are technically overweight. Scientists do this in a much more precise way, using special calipers to measure the width of a fold of skin over the muscles on the back of the upper arm and a fold of skin below the shoulder blade (see Figure 4.4). The first measurement gives a fairly accurate estimate of the fat stored on your limbs, and the second indicates how much fat is stored in your body, usually around your gut and beneath

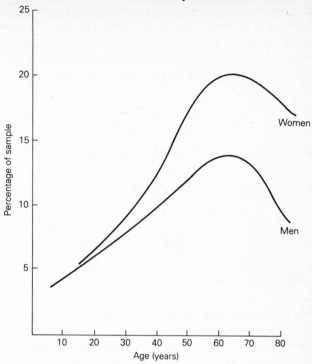

FIG. 4.3. *Obesity in relation to age and sex (UK and Australian data)*

your skin. Taken together the two measurements give a reasonable estimate of your total adipose (or fat-containing) tissue.

At this point a small problem arises. Adipose tissue is not made up entirely of fat. Fat makes up four-fifths of adipose tissue, the balance being water. A second consideration is that energy is released from adipose tissue relatively slowly. If you need energy quickly, you obtain this not from your adipose tissue but from your glycogen–water pool (which we discussed earlier).

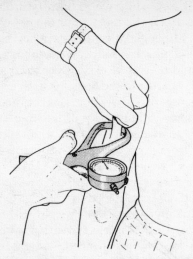

FIG. 4.4. *Measuring skin-fold thickness with calipers*

This is important when a person starves or goes on a very strict weight-reducing diet. If you stay in bed and starve yourself, drinking only water and eating no food, which means that no energy is entering your body, you still need about 7,500 kJ or 1,800 kcal of energy a day to meet the daily energy needs of your body.*

Nearly all of this energy is supplied from the glycogen–water pool, only a small amount being provided by fat stored in the adipose tissue. The glycogen–water pool contains about 17,000 kJ (4,000 kcal) of energy, and will become exhausted after three days of starvation. After this, energy needed for the body to function is obtained by burning fat stored in the adipose tissue.

As 3 kg of water is released from the glycogen–water pool and lost to the body when the 1 kg of glycogen is used up, you will have lost 4 kg of weight. Once your glycogen–water

---

* The actual amount of energy required for your unconscious activities (resting metabolic rate) is not so exact, but the amount of energy required given here is a good approximation.

pool is exhausted, you will have to burn fat from the stores in your adipose tissue to meet your unconscious resting metabolic needs. Although fat contains 37 kJ (9 kcal) of energy per gram, some of this is needed to metabolize the fat to release energy, and only 25 kJ (6 kcal) per gram of fat metabolized is made available to the body for its energy needs. To provide the amount of energy for your resting metabolic needs, you will have to burn 375 g of fat from your adipose tissue each day. In the first week of total starvation you would lose 4 kg from your glycogen–water pool and 1.8 kg from your adipose tissue, a total of 5.8 kg. If you do not remain in bed and continue doing light work, you will use more energy, which is provided from fat stored in your adipose tissue, and a greater loss of weight will occur.

In the second week of complete starvation, when your only energy source is fat obtained from the adipose tissue, only 2.5 kg will be lost. However, it becomes increasingly difficult to starve, and most people start eating again so that the amount of weight lost each week falls progressively.

Rapid weight loss, where the dieter eats a near-starvation diet providing 2,100 kJ (500 kcal), is the basis of many quick-weight-loss diets, but they are effective only for a short period because most people find it hard to keep to a near-starvation diet, and because the water lost from the glycogen–water pool is soon replaced.

The only way to lose weight permanently is to lose it slowly by burning up your fat stores, and this takes time.

If obesity is so common, and if it carries a risk to one's health, why are fat people fat? The answer is not simple. What has been established is that some popular beliefs as to what makes people fat are not true.

One reason for fatness is the wrong choice of parents! Some forms of obesity are due to heredity. This has been shown in several studies. For example, a study that related the parents' (particularly the mother's) size to that of her children showed a close link.

....

Myths about Obesity

The myth	*The fact*
Fat people are lazy.	In general, fat people are as active as thin people.
Fat people absorb food better from their gut.	They do not.
Fat people lack thyroid hormone.	They do not.
Fat people are more addicted to sweet foods than thin people.	They are not.
Obesity is a result of gluttony.	It is not usually.

....

Parents' size	Percentage of children in range (BMI)			
	Underweight	Normal	Overweight	Obese
Overweight	9	39	39	13
Obese	0	40	27	33

The reason for the relationship may be genetic, or because of a similar attitude to food within the family, such as the enjoyment of food, the eating of large meals, snacking between meals, and a lack of physical exercise. In other words, the reason could be environmental rather than genetic. The probability that a genetic factor is the reason was shown in an investigation carried out in Denmark. Scientists followed the progress of people who had been adopted in childhood until they were adult. They found that the weight of the adopted people as adults was much closer to that of their natural parents than to that of their adopted parents. Studies of identical twins carried out over twenty-five years confirm the influence of heredity in obesity.

This raises the question: how does heredity cause obesity? The effect of heredity has been explained by the finding that people prone to obesity use the energy they ingest from food more 'efficiently' than people who have not inherited the

factor for obesity. If you have inherited an 'efficient' metabolism, you will use up less energy for your bodily functions,
and the extra energy obtained from food will be converted
into fat. For example, consider two people, one who has
inherited an 'efficient' metabolism and the other who has
not. They eat the same amount of food each day. The person
who inherited the 'efficient' metabolism will use about 150 kJ
(range 105–270 kJ) less energy each day for bodily functions
than the other. Over a week this adds up about 1,000 kJ
(235 kcal). This amount of energy will make about 28 g (1 oz.)
of fat. (The amount is actually rather less, because the
metabolism of the food uses up some energy, but as an
example it will do.) If this continues for several months, the
'energy-efficient' person will slowly but surely become fat
unless he or she reduces the amount of energy consumed or
takes exercise to lose more of the energy intake. Over a
period of a year the 'energy-efficient' person will gain at least
1 kg more than the other person, and the weight gain will
continue. There is evidence that people who have a strong
genetic trait for obesity do not have spurts of weight gain, as
most of us do, but gain weight steadily over the years. As a
group these people are well adjusted socially; they accept
their body shape and image well, and find it extremely
difficult to lose weight.

Most obese people have a much weaker genetic cause for
their obesity. They may have been slim as children, and may
not have become fat until late adolescence or adulthood.
They can be divided, to some extent, into two groups. The
first group is made up of people who enjoy eating and become fat because they eat too much; in other words, their
obesity is nutritional. The second group is made up of people
who have an eating disorder. They acquire the habit of
overeating to cope with a psychological problem. It is difficult to separate these two groups, and many obese people
probably fit into both groups.

An example of the first group is described by British
scientists who asked nine fat and thirteen lean women to
keep a record of the amount and type of food they ate over

two periods of seven days each. The researchers found that the fat women recorded eating less than the lean women. As the obvious explanation was that the fat women were eating more than they said they ate, the scientists concluded that the fat women had underestimated their food intake and were unable to admit to themselves that it was higher than they believed it to be. In another study, using a sophisticated technique, scientists found that two-thirds of the people they studied habitually underestimated the amount of food they ate.

It is known that many obese people snack between meals and indulge in 'picking' behaviour, eating chocolates, cakes, and sweets at various times during the day. They enjoy a few glasses of beer, or raid the refrigerator for soft drinks. They eat not because they are hungry but because they find eating pleasurable. They do not perceive the snack as food, and having eaten it forget that they have eaten or drunk anything.

If these findings are correct, obesity in some families may be due as much to eating behaviour as to genetic factors. Obese parents may have obese children because the family enjoy food and are big eaters: food and eating are perceived as socially pleasurable and desirable. It is possible that these people are less easily satiated by food, in other words they feel full more slowly. This could be the genetic reason for their obesity, but unfortunately what makes a person feel full after eating a particular amount of food is unknown, so it must remain a theory.

The group of people who have an eating disorder may become obese for the same reasons as the overeaters but, in addition, they tend to overeat or binge-eat when faced with a psychological problem. Their excessive eating is often precipitated by an illness or a disruption to their life. They tend to be slothful, often dependent on others, and sensitive to criticism. They cope with stress, disappointment, a life-crisis, or depression by overeating. If overeating becomes a habit, because the pleasure of food blots out the pain of the problem, the person will gain weight inexorably. In both these groups, habit and learned behaviour may be important in regulating food intake.

Certain diseases cause obesity, but they are rare. Some brain tumours induce obesity, perhaps by affecting the hunger-controlling centre in the brain, as do some uncommon endocrine disorders. In all these conditions, obesity is one of the manifestations of the disease.

Obesity as a Health Hazard

The effect of obesity on health has been investigated by expert committees in several Western countries. Although they differ on detail, these committees have reached the same conclusion. This was expressed succinctly by a study group of the British Medical Association:

We are unanimous in our belief that obesity is a hazard to health and a detriment to well being. It is common enough to constitute one of the most important medical and public health problems of our time, whether we judge importance by a shorter expectation of

....

Obesity and Health Risks

- Diabetes is four times more common in middle-aged obese people than in middle-aged people of normal weight.
- Coronary heart disease is twice as common in obese men under the age of 45.
- High blood pressure and stroke are twice as common in obese people.
- Gall-bladder disease is three times as likely to occur in middle-aged obese women.
- Osteoarthritis, especially of the hips, knees, and back, is more painful and more difficult to relieve if the person is obese.
- Obese women in the reproductive years are more likely to have irregular menstrual periods and to be infertile.
- Very severe obesity (morbid obesity) may cause breathlessness, varicose veins, backache, skin irritation in the fatty folds of skin, and psychological disturbance.

....

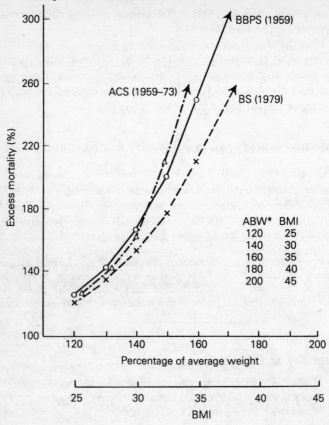

Note: The segments of the lines beyond 140 per cent of average weight in the case of the American Cancer Society (ACS) study and beyond 160 per cent in the Build and Blood Pressure Study (BBPS) and the Build Study (BS) are extrapolations.

* Average body weight

FIG. 4.5. *Excess mortality with obesity*

life, increased morbidity, or cost to the community in terms of both money and anxiety.

Evidence from published studies shows that the more obese the person is the greater his or her chance of dying prematurely (see Figure 4.5).

Obesity also increases the chance that the person will become ill in several ways.

These rather negative findings, however, can be converted to positive findings. If an obese person reduces his or her weight so that the body mass index lies in the normal range, many of these health problems are less likely to occur.

Is Intervention to Treat Obesity Appropriate?

The evidence is that most obese people will be healthier (and perhaps happier) if they lose weight. The problem of intervention to help an obese person reduce weight is that often it is not successful. It requires high motivation and the discipline to adhere to the suggested diet and exercise pro-gramme. Without this motivation and discipline, the amount of weight lost tends to be small when measured over a year.

The problems encountered by an obese person trying to lose weight were stated by a discouraged patient in 1825 in a letter to his physician. He wrote:

Sir, I have followed your prescription as if my life depended upon it, and I have ascertained that during this month I have lost 3 pounds or a little more. But in order to reach this result I have been obliged to do such violence to all my tastes and all my habits—in a word I have suffered so much—that while giving you my best thanks for your kind directions, I renounce the advantages of them and throw myself for the future entirely into the hands or Providence.

Only you can decide if you will follow the weight-reducing regimen or renounce the advantages of losing weight and throw yourself entirely into the hands of Providence. Doctors, dieticians, and nutritionists can help, but in the end a change in eating habits is more important than a weight-reducing programme, and only you can modify those habits. This will be discussed in Chapter 13.

5 ALL FLESH IS AS GRASS: COMPLEX CARBOHYDRATES IN THE DIET

••••••••••••••••••••••••••••••

Most of the food eaten by humans comes from plants: cereals, vegetables, and fruits. Plants consist mainly of complex carbohydrates, which are synthesized from water and carbon dioxide in the air, under the influence of sunlight. Some of the complex carbohydrate is used to make the fibrous tissue which adds strength to the walls of the cells which make up the plant, and helps to keep the plant erect. The rest of the carbohydrate provides the energy the plant requires for growth and any excess is stored in the plant cells in the form of starch or sugar.

Starch is stored in all cereal grains and in roots and tubers such as potato, sweet potato, kumera, and yam. A few plants store sugar, notably sugar cane and sugar beet. When starch is eaten, it is broken down into sugars, mostly glucose, which are absorbed through the gut into the bloodstream. A small amount of the energy absorbed is used immediately, but most is converted either into glycogen (an animal's equivalent of starch) and joins the glycogen–water pool in the muscles, or into fat and stored in the adipose tissue of the body.

If energy is needed quickly, for example because you start strenuous exercise, it is released from the glycogen–water pool rather than from adipose tissue.

As well as supplying energy, plant food supplies dietary

fibre (from the walls of the cells of the plant), vitamins, and minerals. Until recently, dietary fibre was thought to have no nutritional value; now it is thought to be beneficial to health.

If the plant food is boiled, most of the vitamins are destroyed, as they are if the starch is processed and refined to produce white flour, white rice, or sugar. In other words, the complex carbohydrates which made up the plant are converted into simple carbohydrates which are nutritionally less beneficial to health.

The complex carbohydrates obtained from plants are important because they provide most of the energy the human body needs in order to function: to maintain the resting, unconscious body functions; to power the repair and maintenance of its tissues; to provide the energy needed for activity; and to secure a store of energy that is available when food is not.

You may be surprised to know that carbohydrates make up less than 1 per cent of the mass of your body. The amount is small because the complex carbohydrates obtained from food are rapidly burned up or converted into either glycogen to enter the glycogen–water pool or to be stored in the liver, or into triglycerides.

In rich developed countries, carbohydrates in the diet provide about 50 per cent of the total calories eaten each day (see Figure 5.1). In the hungry developing countries, carbohydrates provide up to 70–80 per cent of the energy needed for one day. In all countries, the poorer you are the more cheap carbohydrates and the less expensive protein (and fat) you eat in your diet. There are few exceptions to this. For example, Eskimos eat very few carbohydrates, because, in their environment of snow for most of the year and tundra for the rest, few are available. They have adapted their diet to meet the environment, and eat large quantities of fat instead. In East Africa the Masai tribe lives on foods of mainly animal origin—meat, and milk or blood—and eats very few carbohydrates.

This suggests that carbohydrates are not an essential part of the human diet, but for most people they are a favoured

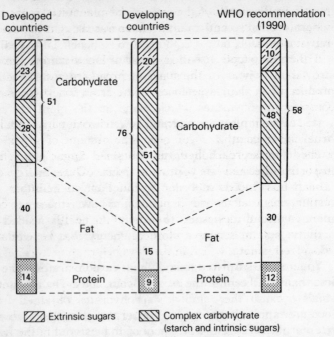

FIG. 5.1. *Composition of diet in developed and developing countries and WHO recommendations (based on amount of energy provided by each component) (%)*

form of food. Humans, with the exceptions I have mentioned, prefer to eat a mixed diet with proteins, fats, and carbohydrates in varying proportions, depending on cultural, economic, and climatic conditions. Most people in most countries obtain most of their energy supply by eating carbohydrates.

The principal form of carbohydrate eaten in the West is based on wheat, and to a lesser extent on potatoes and other root vegetables. Most Asians prefer rice, most Africans eat maize, and Pacific islanders eat tubers such as yams, sweet potatoes, and kumera. With the increasing interchange of cultural information and travel, many of the wealthier people in the developing countries have acquired a taste for wheat products, and many Westeners eat rice as well as wheat products.

For most people living in the developed nations (except for Japan) wheat in the form of bread, breakfast cereals, and pasta is the staple food. These foods are discussed in Chapter 6.

In addition, most people in all countries eat sugar obtained from sugar cane or sugar beet. The amount of sugar consumed varies greatly between countries. Sugar is a refined carbohydrate, and has been called 'pure, white, and deadly'. This phrase exaggerates the harmful effects of sugar, but emphasizes that too much sugar in the diet instead of complex carbohydrates is not beneficial to health. As well as being a palatable source of energy, sugar has benefits as a food preservative, which in the days before snap freezing and refrigeration enabled people living in cold countries to eat a more varied diet in the winter months. Sugar is discussed in Chapter 7.

Another component of plants is what nutritionists call non-starch polysaccharide, or dietary fibre. It is only relatively recently that the value of fibre in the diet has been appreciated. Dietary fibre is discussed in Chapter 8.

6 OUR DAILY BREAD

• •

> If I am hungry...I don't care whether the bread is
> black, brown, or white. My stomach wants to be filled,
> not entertained.
>
> Seneca

About 40,000 years ago humankind learned how to make fire,
and 30,000 years later how to cultivate grasses whose seeds
they had previously only picked. By judicious selection or,
more likely, by trial and error, they began the conscious
cultivation of barley and wheat. They gathered the barley
seeds, pounded them, and made porridge of the result by
cooking the pounded cereals. This astonishing advance in
food technology was first practised in the foothills of the
Tigris–Euphrates valley in Asia Minor, and spread as the
nomadic tribes moved further afield. But porridge was relatively unsatisfying. It had to be eaten when it was cooked,
and it was difficult to carry. By 2000 BC flat unleavened cakes
of flour were replacing porridge, and wheat was gradually
replacing barley. The wheaten cakes kept fairly well after
cooking and could be eaten later. This was not possible with
barley meal. But this time, the naked wheats, which are
more suitable for bread-making, had largely displaced the
husked, or emmer, wheat of earlier times. It is likely that
emmer wheat had been used to make unleavened bread,
especially for ritual occasions, and the husking was probably
effected by burning off the ears. This process is suggested by
the reference in the Bible, in the Book of Ruth, to 'parched
corn'.

By Graeco-Roman times both a hard and a soft wheat had
been developed, the latter making the most palatable bread.

But the process of making this white bread was time-consuming and expensive, and so it was a luxury reserved for the rich. At the same time a coarse wholemeal bread was made, which had known laxative properties. Since it would be inhospitable to offer such bread to guests, wealthy people of high social status served their guests with bread made from fine flour, and white bread became a status symbol. It was probably produced by sieving a well-ground wheaten flour, which separated the flour from the bran and the sand that had been added to the grind mix to help remove the husks.

With the expansion of the Roman Empire, wheaten bread became the staple cereal food in the Mediterranean area, and this Roman preference was to persist throughout Europe for over 2,000 years. In England, for example, in AD 1206, the Assize of Bread was established to prevent speculation in flour and excessive fluctuations in the price of bread. The legislation laid down how millers' and bakers' charges, and the retail price of bread, should vary with the cost of the grain. The usual bread was made from wheat, although rye and other cereals were also grown, mainly to provide food for animals. Barley was grown principally for brewing beer, and it was eaten by the poor. In other northern European countries rye bread was as important a food as wheaten bread. But even in these countries, the richer families chose white wheaten bread.

For 500 years the Bread Assizes in England controlled the price of bread, recognizing three grades: white, wheaten, and household. The white flour was reserved for the feudal families, and was baked in small loaves (like dinner rolls) weighing about 200 g each. They were soft in texture and white in colour. The lesser gentry ate a loaf weighing about 500 g, which was made of whole wheat from which the coarse bran had been sieved. The poor and the servants ate a coarse loaf in which wheat wholemeal, rye, and barley flour were mixed. This was known as household bread. The long period during which bread was graded and controlled confirmed in the minds of the English that white bread was a superior food, softer and more palatable, and with the rise of the mercantile classes it became a status symbol to have white bread on the table. There was also a belief that wholemeal bread caused diarrhoea, which could be lethal, especially in children. Probably the laxative effects of wholemeal bread were confused with the deadly symptoms of typhoid and other enteric diseases. Furthermore, wholemeal bread resembled oatmeal, which was eaten by the despised Scots. (The poor of England also rejected the potato as a substitute for bread, as it was used for animal feed, and was eaten by the dirty, decadent, papist Irish.)

The belief that white bread was superior to brown, that it was nutritionally better, tasted better, and to be preferred, was a long-lasting cultural tradition, but despite popular belief, no objective, scientific investigations had been made to confirm or deny the superiority of white bread over brown. Some people dissented from the popular view. They were mostly intellectuals, usually had good incomes, and were generally regarded as cranks. De Quincey, the self-confessed opium addict, perhaps typifies them and their views. In a letter to a friend, inviting him to stay at Wordsworth's house in Grasmere, De Quincey wrote, 'I would offer you some temptations ... mountain lamb ... trout and pike ... bread, such as you have never presumed to dream of, made of our own wheat, not doctored and separated by the usual miller's process into insipid flour, and coarse—that is merely dirty-looking white, but all ground down together, which is the sole receipt of having rich, lustrous, red-brown ambrosial bread.'

To the average Englishman, De Quincey's views were suspect, his prose too ethereal and his tastes too exotic. What an Englishman and his family wanted was good, fresh, spongy, white bread.

J H, who is otherwise unnamed, wrote in a letter as 'Advocate for Public Welfare' in 1773, 'On the occasion of the public enquiry concerning the most fit and proper bread to be assized for general use': 'The prejudices of the people are strong; but they relate chiefly to the magic of the two syllables *white* and *brown*.'

The magic of these two syllables has persisted until today, but now there is scientific evidence on which to base the decision whether to eat white bread or brown.

The scientific assessment of the nutritive values of brown and white bread remained a dream until 1945 because of the ethical impossibility of performing a feeding experiment on humans. Then, in the aftermath of the most destructive war in history, undernutrition was the lot of many Europeans, particularly the Germans. In these circumstances, the Department of Experimental Medicine at Cambridge University suggested to the Medical Research Council that it would be ethically possible to set up an experimental feeding scheme, under the direction of Professor R. A. McCance.

In the town of Wuppertal in the state of Westphalia, Germany, there was a home for abandoned children, aged 5 to 15. In 1947 food was in short supply, and examination showed that the children were shorter and lighter than American children of corresponding ages. In fact they weighed 9 per cent less and were 5 per cent shorter than their American counterparts. The plan was that in addition to the food rations available, the children would be divided into five groups, each of which would be given a different kind to bread. They would be encouraged to eat as much bread as they liked. The five breads were made of wholemeal flour; 85 per cent flour; 70 per cent flour enriched with vitamins and iron to the concentration found in wholemeal; 70 per cent flour with vitamins and iron in the concentration found in 85 per cent extracted flour; and finally bread made of 70 per cent unenriched flour. The children were carefully examined at the start of the feeding programme, and received supplements of calcium and vitamins A, C, and D throughout the experiment. They were to be examined again from time to time and tested for levels of protein, vitamins of the B complex, and iron, for these nutrients were known to be removed during milling.

Once the breads were available, the children fell on this extra windfall like ravenous wolves. Quite soon they were all getting about 70 per cent of their energy from bread. In addition they had soups, potatoes, and vegetables, but meat and eggs were very scarce, providing only about 8 g of protein a day.

Professor McCance argued that 'with such a high proportion of bread in their diets, and so little protective foods, everything possible had been done to bring out the differences in the nutritional value of the breads', and the differences would show up quite quickly. In fact, no differences appeared. The children in each of the five groups began to improve at an equal rate. At the end of the year there were still no differences, but by now the children had heights and weights comparable to their American counterparts.

After this experience, Professor McCance and his colleagues studied other groups of children and also began feeding experiments on young rats. In 1951 and 1954 the results of their work were published in two special reports by the Medical Research Council of Great Britain. These reports made it clear that, following the field experiments in feeding German children, and the laboratory experiments in feeding rats, it was 'most improbable that nutritional differences between one bread, or another, would ever be demonstrated in children whether they were well-nourished or under-nourished', even when the rest of their diet contained only small quantities of milk, animal protein, or other 'protective' foods, such as vitamins and trace elements. But the reports confirmed the importance of having some of the protective foods in every diet.

What the scientists ignored was that white bread had only about one-third the amount of dietary fibre contained in the equivalent quantity of wholemeal bread. At that time the importance of dietary fibre was not appreciated. Today fibre is added to many white breads, because most people still prefer white bread to brown.

To the general public, white bread still has a status value: when fresh it is spongier, it looks cleaner, and many think it tastes better. Millers prefer white flour because they can produce it more cheaply than brown, they believe that they can sell more bread by adding improvers to make the bread still whiter. They can also make use of the 20 per cent residue left after milling white flour. This is the bran that is sold for animal food, or as the wheat bran sold in pharmacies. Bakers prefer white bread because it is easier to mould the dough and bake the bread in today's mechanized bakeries.

Opposed to this trend are two groups who advocate wholemeal bread. The first and most vocal group today are those who want a return to a more organic type of food, a food in which no chemicals have been used during growth, and no additives used in processing. They reject much of the artificiality of modern life, and seek a simpler more 'natural' existence. The second group is made up of those who believe that the consumption over the years of white flour may damage their health, because their diet lacks dietary fibre. (These matters are discussed in greater detail in Chapter 8.) It must be stated, however, that bread made from white flour does contain some fibre (3 g per 100 g of bread), although this is one-third the amount in wholemeal bread, as do many breakfast cereals.

7 SUGAR AND SPICE AND ALL THINGS NICE

• •

> What are little girls made of?
> What are little girls made of?
> Sugar and spice and all things nice:
> That's what little girls are made of.
>
> Nursery rhyme

The sugar we eat includes the sugar that is incorporated into the structure of our foods (intrinsic sugars), the sugar that occurs in milk and milk products, and that (usually sucrose) obtained by refining sugar cane or sugar beet (refined or non-milk extrinsic sugar).

In the past 175 years the consumption of refined sugar in Western countries has risen spectacularly. In England in the late 1700s a person ate on average 10 kg of refined sugar a year. One hundred years later the average consumption had risen to 30 kg a year, and in 1990 an average person in England and Wales and in Australia was eating 35 kg a year, that is about 95 g (3⅓ oz.) of refined sugar a day. This amount represents a decrease over the past twenty years. In the USA the rise in consumption of refined sugar has been similar, but an average American eats only four-fifths as much sugar as is eaten by a Briton or an Australian. The quantity of sugar eaten also differs according to the age of the person. Both in Britain and in the USA, young children are the greatest sugar-eaters, boys eating rather more than girls.

Most of the refined sugar consumed is obtained from sugar added to cereals and soft drinks, or in confectionery, jams,

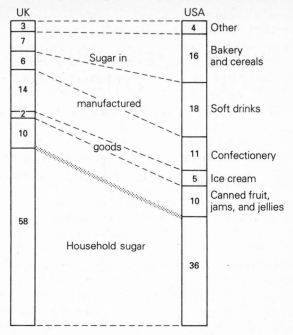

FIG. 7.1. *Sugar eaten in the home in the UK and the USA (%)*

cakes, and biscuits. There is a difference in the type of sugar-rich foods eaten in Britain and the USA, although the difference is diminishing. In simple terms, Americans eat more ice cream and drink more soft drinks than the British, who eat more household sugar and confectionery than Americans (Figure 7.1).

The increase in refined-sugar consumption started in the eighteenth century when cane sugar from the Caribbean became readily available in Britain and the USA, and coincided with changes in diet as the countries grew richer. With increasing affluence people eat more meat, more saturated fats and oils, more total fat, and more sugar, and less vegetables, cereals, potatoes (and other tubers) than people in poor countries. By contrast, most people living in the developing countries eat little meat, their diet consisting to a large extent of complex carbohydrate, vegetables, and fruits, with some sugar.

In the past fifty years, food choices have increased dramatically, and prepackaged 'convenience' foods and sugar-rich drinks have become readily available. Within a country, people who have more disposable income change their diet more than the poor, but the dietary changes are found among all classes in the society. Some of the dietary changes that have occurred in England and Wales since 1770 are shown below (in terms of kilograms per head per year):

	1770	1870	1990
Sugar	10	30	35
Potatoes	44	146	87
Bread (wheat flour)	180	137	73
Fats	9	27	59

Most people in Western countries are surprised, or even indignant, when they are told that they eat 35 kg of sugar a year. This is because only 30 per cent of the sugar consumed is visible, that is, it is used to sweeten breakfast cereals, tea, and coffee. The rest, which may include high-fructose corn syrup, is 'hidden' in cakes, biscuits, pastries, jams, ice cream, confectionery, chocolates (which also contain fat), canned fruits, and soft drinks or mixer drinks. A small amount of sugar (in the form of fructose) is also contained in most fresh fruits. Hidden sugar accounts for 70 per cent of the daily intake, and amounts to nearly 60 g (2 oz.)!

In most developed countries legislation has been passed which makes it obligatory for food manufacturers to display the ingredients of the food on the package, and in some cases the quantities of the ingredients, including the amount of sugar 'hidden' in the product. However, most people do not read the label, and hence do not know how much sugar they are eating in the manufactured food.

In the developed countries of the world, between 15 and 25 per cent of the energy eaten each day is in the form of sugar,

although, as mentioned, the proportion is beginning to fall—slowly.

Sugar has been described as made up of 'empty' calories, the implication being that it contains only energy, and provides no minerals, vitamins, or protein to the consumer.

In fact, sugar, that is sucrose, honey, and corn syrup, is the only food eaten by humans that supplies no nutrients whatsoever.

Some health fanatics deny this and claim that only white sugar lacks nutrients. They are wrong. Raw sugar, honey, and corn syrup are as devoid of nutrients as white sugar. They provide energy but no protein, vitamins, or minerals needed to keep your body healthy. Refined sugar is 99.9 per cent pure sucrose; honey is 99 per cent fructose (which tastes sweeter than sucrose); and raw sugar is 96 per cent sucrose (and 3 per cent fibre).

The more sugar replaces complex carbohydrates in the diet, the less nutritious is the diet.

There are several good reasons why people in affluent countries eat so much sugar. Sugar, because it is sweet, helps form our concept of what is palatable in food. Palatability is defined as the subjective qualities of food: its texture, its colour, its taste, and its smell or absence of smell. White sugar looks good, it has a clean texture, and most important of all it tastes good. So does honey, which is sweeter than sugar and has, in addition, the emotional value that it is natural and therefore must be wholesome, and that it was the sweetener used long before sugar became available.

Most humans are conditioned to like sweet foods if they are readily available. People have a sweet tooth. Children are rewarded for being good by being given sweet foods. Even if parents limit the amount of sweet food that a pre-school child eats, once the child is at school peer pressure could induce him or her to choose and to eat sweet foods, which are enjoyable and taste good.

There are good reasons why manufacturers use sugar. First, it makes foods palatable, which increases sales. Second, sugar has valuable preservative properties. Added to jams, jellies, preserves, and condensed milk, it reduces the chance of bacterial growth by its moisture-removing properties. Sugar added to ice-cream helps the mixture to freeze more rapidly. In bread- and cake-making, sugar is needed to make the yeast rapidly produce the carbon dioxide necessary for the raising effect that creates the airy texture in bread which people enjoy. Sugar also forms a complex with the gluten in the flour which helps the gluten to expand, producing a light-textured cake or bread. However, in bread-making, the amount of sugar does not add to a person's sucrose intake, as it is all used up in the bread-making process.

Is there any harm in eating the amount of sugar we eat in the developed countries? Twenty years ago scientists believed that excess intake of sugar over the years might be a cause of a form of diabetes (non-insulin-dependent diabetes mellitus, NIDDM) which usually started in middle age and was becoming increasingly common. Another common disorder, dental decay (caries) was also thought to be associated with diets that contained a large amount of sugar. The third health problem in which sugar was thought to be implicated was the development of obesity. What is the truth about these beliefs?

Diabetes and Diet

There are two types of diabetes. The first is insulin-dependent diabetes mellitus (IDDM), which is thought to be an autoimmune disorder, in which the insulin-secreting cells in the pancreas are destroyed by the body's own cells. IDDM starts in childhood or early adolescence and is due to a lack of insulin, as the insulin-secreting cells are unable to supply enough to regulate glucose metabolism in the body. Insulin controls the level of sugar in the blood, and plays a key role in maintaining glucose supplies to the tissues. If this control is lost, serious complications result. A person who has IDDM requires regular injections of insulin to avoid becoming very ill, or even dying. Control of glucose levels by insulin also helps to avoid the chronic effects of IDDM, that is, damage to small blood vessels, which leads to blindness, patches of gangrene on the feet or legs, impotence, and severe kidney disease. The proportion of people who have IDDM is higher in developed than in developing countries, but even in developed countries IDDM accounts for only 10 per cent of all cases of diabetes.

The second type of diabetes is non-insulin-dependent diabetes mellitus (NIDDM). In NIDDM insulin continues to be secreted, often in insufficient amounts, because of damage to the insulin-secreting cells of the pancreas, and even when the normal amount is secreted the body is unable to use the hormone effectively. NIDDM starts later in life, usually after the age of 35. Between 3 and 6 per cent of the adult population of most Western developed countries have NIDDM, and the prevalence of the disease increases with advancing age.

In developed countries most of the people who have NIDDM are overweight or obese. This suggests that obesity and diabetes are in some way connected. Among people from the developing countries who have NIDDM, only a quarter are overweight or obese, and so, in their case, factors other than obesity must be involved in the onset of the disease. This suggests that diet predisposes some people, who have a low tolerance to carbohydrate, to NIDDM. What has not been established is whether it is excessive energy intake, or the excessive intake of simple carbohydrate (sugar and white flour) or fat, or both, that plays the main role. Current opinion supports the view that excessive energy intake from both carbohydrate and fat, rather than from either alone, is related to NIDDM, but a low content of fibre in the diet and a lack of exercise are probably additional factors.

The most persuasive evidence that life-style and diet are involved in the development of NIDDM is that it is becoming increasingly prevalent among people in developing countries, and native people in developed countries, who abandon their traditional life-style and diet to adopt a 'Western'-style of life.

In North America, before they were dispossessed of their lands by white Americans and resettled on reservations, native Americans ate maize in large quantities, and hunted and gathered their food. On the reservations, they were given hand-outs of white flour and sugar. The change of diet, and the lack of physical activity led to health problems: they became fat and developed diabetes, which now affects three or four times as many native Americans as other Americans.

In Australia, before white settlement, the native Koori derived most of their food from roots and vegetables, supplemented by meat when the hunters were successful. Within a hundred years of white settlement, most Kooris were living on reservations. They took little exercise and received hand-outs of tea, white flour, and sugar. The change in their life-style and diet (they also began to consume alcohol) resulted in obesity, diabetes, and heart disease—which are three to four times more common among Koori than among white Australians.

In Zimbabwe rural Africans, whose diet consists mostly of maize, and little fat and sugar, have a low incidence of NIDDM. Urban Africans, in contrast, who have changed to a different life-style and whose diet has become more 'Westernized', with greater consumption of fats and sugar, are increasingly being diagnosed as having NIDDM.

Pakistani and Indian immigrants to the United Kingdom in the years after the Second World War, who also changed their diet, from one mainly of wheat flour in the form of chapattis, or rice, towards a more typical British diet, now have an incidence of diabetes three times that among white British people. The change in diet cannot be the whole explanation, however, as studies in India have found that the incidence of NIDDM among urban Indians is also high.

In the twenty years after the Second World War, Pacific islanders increasingly chose to change from their traditional life-style and diet to a 'Western' life-style and diet, and began to develop NIDDM.

A theory to explain the increase in NIDDM (and other 'diseases of affluence' such as high blood pressure and coronary heart disease) was developed in 1962. This was the 'thrifty gene' theory, which proposes as follows: Before contact with Europeans, most indigenous races had an uncertain food supply because their source of food could be, and often was, eliminated by hurricanes or droughts. They alternated between periods of good food supply (feasts) and famines. Those whose metabolism favoured the accumulation of fat in their bodies when food was plentiful had a survival advantage during the famines, in other words their genes were programmed to cope with the alternating pattern of available food. With the change to a 'Western' life-style and diet, famines became almost unknown, and most days were feast days (although non-traditional types of food were usually eaten). When the people had an abundance of food each day, particularly foods rich in fats or based on refined flour, and were given quantities of sugar, they tended to become fat and engaged less in physical activity. The foods also contained far less fibre than they had obtained from their traditional diet. The gene that was useful in the days when feast and famine alternated now became potentially dangerous. In the person who had this 'thrifty gene', the dietary and life-style changes resulted in progressive damage to the pancreatic beta cells, which led in time to NIDDM.

All these studies suggest that a lethargic life-style and a diet that provides an excessive amount of energy, particularly from fat and sugar, and little fibre, may predispose susceptible people to develop non-insulin-dependent diabetes, and that a change in diet and the taking of physical exercise may prevent the disease occurring in many of them.

There is some evidence for this. A group of diabetic Koori were induced to go back for a few weeks to a traditional hunter–gatherer life-style. During this period their NIDDM disappeared. Studies by Professor Paul Zimmet, to whom I am indebted for the information in this section, have shown that among male Pacific islanders and Mauritians who have an active life-style, the prevalence of NIDDM is about half that of the inactive males.

These studies suggest that the dietary change to a high-energy Western-style diet, rather than an excess of sugar, is the main reason for the increasing prevalence of NIDDM in developing countries.

Dental Caries

Until recently, dietary sugar was a major factor in the second health problem, dental caries. Dietary sugar still causes dental problems in countries or parts of countries where the drinking water is not fluoridated.

The effect of diet on the health of the teeth is demonstrated by an investigation made in 1960 by a British dental surgeon, Professor Hardwick. He examined over 1,000 teeth in skulls, which carbon-dating had established as belonging to people living in the sixth century AD. He compared the teeth with the teeth of people living in 1960. Dental caries occurred in only 9.5 per cent of the Anglo-Saxon teeth, whose diet consisted of complex carbohydrates, vegetables, and a small amount of meat. The people living in 1960, whose diet was rich in sugar and fats, were found to have dental caries affecting 48.5 per cent of their teeth.

The amount of sugar in the diet is a major factor in the development of tooth decay. This is demonstrated by studies in Britain and Scandinavia during the Second World War. During the war years, and for some time afterwards, sugar and manufactured foods based on sugar, such as sweets, chocolates, cakes, and biscuits, were rationed in most European countries. To replace these foods, people ate more bread, potatoes, and vegetables. It was found that during these years the number of children with tooth decay showed a steady progressive decline. After 1948, when sugar became readily available again, the prevalence of dental caries began to rise, until halted by fluoridation of drinking water, after which the prevalence of dental caries has declined dramatically.

The effect of sugar, in the form of sweet drinks, among children whose drinking water is fluoridated has been shown recently. In New South Wales dentists have reported more dental decay in the milk-teeth of children who are given sweet drinks than in other children.

Why does Dental Caries Occur?

Teeth are composed mainly of a tough bone called dentine, over which is a thin coat of enamel, which is the hardest tissue in the body. Inside the dentine is the tooth pulp, which contains nerves and blood vessels. Dental decay begins when particles of food containing sugar stick on to the surface of the teeth, or become impacted into the normal crevices of the tooth's structure. The food particles, together with saliva and the myriads of bacteria that are always in the mouth, form a small plaque, rather like a miniature cow-pat, which sticks tightly on to the tooth's surface. There are two main kinds of bacteria in the plaque. They are called streptococci and lactobacilli. The streptococci convert any sugars in the food (but preferentially convert sucrose) into a complex carbohydrate substance called dextran. The dextran is relished by the lactobacilli, which release an acid as they grow and multiply. The acid is produced in the plaque of food as it adheres to the tooth, and since it is not neutralized by the alkaline saliva, gradually eats into the dentine through cracks in the enamel.

The clinical observations reported earlier, and experimental studies on rats, confirm that sucrose in the diet plays a significant part in causing dental caries, unless the teeth are protected by fluoride, which makes the enamel more resistant to plaque. In areas where water is not treated with fluoride, dental caries can be reduced if you avoid snacks of sugary food, and clean your teeth after eating.

Sugar and Obesity

Obesity has been discussed in Chapter 4, where it was explained that if energy intake regularly exceeds energy expenditure, people will inevitably become overweight and eventually obese. It was also noted that foods rich in fat, and sugary foods, are implicated in the development of obesity. Fats provide more energy (25 kJ or 6 kcal per gram) than sugar (17 kJ or 4 kcal per gram), so fatty foods make you feel full more quickly than sugary foods, such as confectionery, soft drinks, or tea or coffee with added sugar. Hence sugary foods tend to encourage you to continue snacking. It is quite

....

How to Cut Down on Sugar

- Start by cutting down the number of spoons of sugar you add to your cup of tea or coffee, and over a few weeks cut out all sugar you use in hot drinks. What you are doing is desensitizing your taste buds' demand for a sweet taste.
- If you eat breakfast cereals or porridge, sprinkle as little sugar as you can on it, or preferably use no sugar, honey, or syrup.
- Avoid eating cakes and sweet biscuits, except on special occasions.
- Cut out ordinary soft drinks; drink low-calorie ones instead, which contain non-nutritive sweeteners and no sugar. The new non-nutritive sweeteners, such as aspartame, appear to be safe to eat.
- Better still, buy citrus fruit and make your own fruit drink instead. The fructose in the fruit will make it sweet enough and you will not need to add sucrose.
- If you drink alcohol, choose the lighter (less sugary) varieties of beer and avoid ginger ale, bitter lemon, and tonic in your brandy or gin. The first is very sweet; the others seem to be bitter, but in reality are loaded with hidden sugar.
- Stop eating sweets, chocolates, and toffees between meals. If you need to chew something, chew an apple!
- But don't be obsessive. If you want to eat a cake or a piece of chocolate or some ice-cream, or drink a soft drink from time to time, you can!

....

easy to eat 300 to 400 g of sugar a day, which will provide 5,000–6,700 kJ (1,200–1,600 kcal) of energy, without realizing how much energy you are absorbing.

Because of the effect of sugary foods on the development of dental caries, but more particularly because of its involvement in the development of obesity, several expert committees have recommended that the amount of sugar consumed by people in developed countries should be reduced by up to 50 per cent. These recommendations apply particularly to the 30 per cent of the adult population who are overweight or obese.

There are problems in achieving this dietary goal. Sugar is sweet and tastes good. If the habit of eating sugar starts early in life, it is hard to break it. Manufacturers of breakfast cereals and confectionery are well aware that children have a sweet tooth, and seek to pander to a child's desire for new, novel confectionery. Parents and relatives may try to counter the persuasive advertising by rewarding a child with fresh fruit or a sugar-free drink rather than sweets or biscuits. But the success rate is low!

8 THE NOT SO USELESS FIBRE

· ·

Fibre is the most successful buzz word today.
Food Processing Magazine (1990)

Fibre is the part of a plant that makes the wall of cells and provides the plant with solidity and stiffness. Until recently, fibre was thought to have no value. It is now known that dietary fibre, the remnant of the cell wall eaten in food, is of considerable value for health.

Dietary fibre is no more an 'it' than are vitamins. There are many kinds of fibre, but all of them are made up from long chains of sugars, and are described as non-starch polysaccharides. Some plant fibres are soluble, which means that they form thick solutions (gels) when mixed with water. Others are insoluble, which means that they pass through the gut unaltered.

Soluble dietary fibre includes guar gum and pectin, and a group of fibres with exotic names (ispaghula, xanthan, betaglucans), which seem to be laxatives, possibly by stimulating the cells that line the gut. Soluble dietary fibres affect the body by their actions in the stomach and small bowel. They reduce the rate of stomach-emptying and of small-bowel motility. This may reduce the rise in blood glucose and insulin concentrations that normally occurs after a meal (and in this way may be of benefit in controlling diabetes), and regulate blood cholesterol to some extent.

Insoluble dietary fibre, which makes up the stringy or woody parts of plants, include cellulose, lignin, and aribinoxylans, speeds up the transit of food through the gut, increases the bulk of the faeces, and is an effective laxative.

The belief that fibre might have a health value was first suggested in 1880 in England, by Dr Allison, who believed that constipation was 'one great curse of this country, which is caused in great measure by [eating] white bread. From constipation come piles, varicose veins, headaches, miserable feelings, dullness and other ailments.' He suggested that constipation could be cured by eating bread made from 100 per cent wholemeal flour, which of course contained dietary fibre.

Dr Allison's belief that many 'Western diseases' were due to a deficiency of fibre in the diet was revived in 1969 by Dr Denis Burkitt and Dr T. L. Cleave. Dr Burkitt had practised medicine in Africa for many years and Dr Cleave had been to many parts of the world during his time in the Royal Navy. The two doctors observed, independently, that people in developed countries seemed to contract certain diseases which were unusual in the countries of the developing world. As many of the diseases were related to the intestinal tract, they wondered if the diet eaten by people in Western countries might be the reason for their increased incidence. They then explored the changes that have occurred in the British diet in the past hundred years.

Since the last quarter of the nineteenth century very considerable changes have taken place in the British diet. In about 1870 steel rollers replaced the traditional stones for grinding flour. The steel rollers separated the husk from the flour more efficiently than the traditional grinding stones, so that greater quantities of white flour became available at a reduced cost, enabling more people to choose the whiter breads with lower extraction rates. In 1870 a person ate on average about 400 g of bread per day, together with 300 g of potatoes, and vegetables and a little fruit. This diet yielded about 40 g of dietary fibre, about 8 g of which was crude fibre, mainly from cereals.

Since 1870 the average consumption of bread in England has fallen to 200 g (7 oz.) a day, and most people choose to eat white bread, which contains 1 g of fibre per slice, rather than wholemeal bread, which contains 2.5 g of fibre per slice. Over the same period, the consumption of potatoes has also fallen to 240 g (8½ oz.) a day, and more fats and sugar are eaten each day.

In 1870 sugar and fats (to a lesser extent) contributed about 25 per cent of a person's daily energy supply. Today our consumption of refined carbohydrates (and of fats to a lesser extent) has increased, so that these two nutrients provide over 50 per cent of our daily energy intake.

These dietary changes have resulted in a considerable fall in the amount of dietary fibre we consume each day—from about 40 g a day in 1870 to about 20 g a day in 1990.

One major effect of the change of diet, according to Dr Burkitt, has been to alter the behaviour of our intestinal tracts and to prolong the time it takes for food to pass through the body. With the aid of colleagues in South Africa and London, Dr Burkitt examined the transit times of stools in various groups of people eating different diets. To do this, volunteers swallowed twenty-five radio-opaque pellets the size of rice grains, and collected the next five or six stools into plastic bags. By this simple method, the investigators were able to determine how long it took the pellets to pass through the gut, and to relate the transit time to the size of the stool. The groups of volunteers who ate a refined, low-fibre diet were British naval ratings and their wives, teenage British boarding-school students, and white university students in South Africa. The groups that ate a mixed diet, with a moderate amount of fibre, were hospital patients in England, Indian nurses in South Africa, urban African schoolchildren, English vegetarians, and Ugandan African boarding-school students. The groups that ate a high-fibre diet were rural schoolchildren in South Africa and rural villagers in Uganda.

When the results were analysed, Dr Burkitt found that the more fibre there was in the diet, the bulkier the stool was and the faster the bulky soft stool was propelled through the bowel. This was true whether the person was a rural Ugandan villager or a vegetarian English vicar. Those who had a high fibre content in their diet had similar bowel habits; the transit time was about 40 hours, and the stool weighed over 300 g. In contrast, the people who ate a traditional English diet, with a low fibre and high sugar content, had daily stools weighing about 110 g, and a transit time of 80 hours. It was interesting that when bran was added to the traditional English diet, the bulk of the stool increased nearly to that of the English vegetarian's, and the transit time diminished.

Dr Burkitt's work, and that of the other investigators, confirms that diets containing a higher amount of fibre result in large quantities of soft stools that pass through the intestine quickly. But the refined, low-fibre diets favoured in developed countries produce small, firm stools that linger in the bowel for a long time. No wonder the British are so obsessed with their bowel function, and resort so readily to laxatives!

A number of diseases seem to be characteristic of developed Western nations but are rarely encountered in the developing countries. One group of these diseases, commonly found in Western civilizations, are bowel, or gastro-intestinal, diseases. Heart disease is also more common in developed countries, and a lack of dietary fibre may be involved.

The Gastro-Intestinal Diseases

The gastro-intestinal diseases which are frequently found in developed Western countries but are less common in developing countries are constipation, haemorrhoids, appendicitis, irritable bowel syndrome, diverticular disease, and colon cancer. The role of lack of fibre in the diet in causing constipation and haemorrhoids is accepted by most scientists. There is less unanimity about the role of dietary fibre in the other four disorders.

The Not So Useless Fibre

Constipation

Dietary fibre increases the bulk of the stool in two ways. First, it absorbs water so that the stool becomes bulky, and second, it may stimulate the cells lining the gut to start contracting. This means, as Dr Burkitt found, that the stool passes more rapidly through the gut, and constipation is relieved.

Cancer of the Large Bowel

The more rapid transit of the stool through the gut may have another beneficial effect. Bile salts are released by the gall-bladder into the gut to help digestion. If the transit time is slow, the millions of bacteria that inhabit the gut act on the bile salts, breaking down the excess not used in digesting foods to form a substance called deoxycholate. The slower transit time of the stools through the intestines permits more deoxycholate to be produced. This may have sinister consequences, as deoxycholate is a cancer-inducing substance in certain people.

Bowel cancer usually occurs in people who have pre-existing bowel polyps, which readily absorb deoxycholate. Over time the polyps may become 'pre-malignant'. If this change is detected, surgery to remove the affected part of the bowel is recommended. The non-affected part is then stitched to the rectum. It is known that polyps are likely to recur in the previously unaffected rectum, and may become cancerous.

A study in the USA has shown that if the people who have had the operation eat fibre-containing foods in amounts sufficient to double their fibre intake, their chance of the cancerous polyps recurring is much reduced. The study did not show whether increased amounts of dietary fibre would prevent the pre-malignant polyps from developing, or whether vegetables were as protective as bran (which is what the scientists used as a source of fibre).

There is a twist to the story. Other scientists have suggested that the increased chance of a Western person developing bowel cancer is due to the increased amount of fat in the Western diet, rather than to a lack of fibre.

Cancer of the large bowel is the most frequently found cancer in middle-aged people in several Western countries, about one person in twenty-five developing it during their lifetime, but it is almost unknown in east and southern Africa. The reason for the difference may be the difference in diet, and dietary fibre may be an important factor. A recent analysis of published papers reported in the *Journal of the National Cancer Institute* provides strong evidence that vegetables and dietary fibre are protective against cancer.

Until the matter is settled about the relative roles of fat (as a factor causing bowel cancer) and dietary fibre and vegetables (as a factor preventing bowel cancer), a wise person might decide to eat extra vegetables, and cereals with added fibre, and to make sure that the amount of dietary fibre eaten is 30 g a day, nearly twice the average amount most people eat.

Haemorrhoids

Haemorrhoids affect between 10 and 20 per cent of all adults in Western countries, and by the age of 50 more than one-third of all adults have haemorrhoids. Haemorrhoids are more common in people who suffer from constipation, which is a consequence of a lack of fibre in the diet.

When a person tries to evacuate a firm, constipated stool, a great deal of effort is needed. This is achieved by fixing the diaphragm, taking a deep breath, and tightening the abdominal muscles. The result is that the intra-abdominal pressure is raised to an astonishing degree. This increase is repeated until eventually the stool is expelled, or the struggle is abandoned for that day.

Each time the abdominal pressure is raised, the pressure increases in the three 'cushions' of veins and muscle that lie just inside your anus, which assist in keeping the faeces inside your bowel until you want to defecate. The result of repeated efforts to expel a firm, constipated stool raises the pressure in the veins, which eventually dilate because their walls are unable to cope with the strain. These dilated veins become varicosities and often prolapse. The result is haemorrhoids, or piles.

One of the factors leading to varicose veins may be the way in which we empty our bowels. In contrast to the majority of the people in the world, we sit rather than squat when we defecate. When you squat to defecate, the direction of the force of the raised intra-abdominal pressure is down into your pelvis directly along the line of the lowest portion of your gut. When you sit to defecate much of the force is transmitted down your legs, raising the pressure within your leg veins.

Your leg veins have valves in them to prevent such pressure causing harm, but if these valves are not very efficient, or are constantly put under pressure, they may stretch, leading to increased pressure in the veins and later distension of the veins themselves. Varicose veins develop.

It is interesting to observe that societies who eat a traditional diet that contains a good deal of fibre rarely suffer from varicose veins: fewer than 2 per cent of the adult population are affected. However, in the affluent nations between 10 and 20 per cent of adults have varicose veins.

The effect of the raised intra-abdominal pressure upwards, not downwards, may account for the increase in hernias of the diaphragm. These are called hiatus hernias. Hiatus hernia is an uncomfortable disorder which becomes increasingly common with advancing age. In affluent, overfed countries routine barium-meal examinations have shown that about 20 per cent of men and 35 per cent of women have the condition. In the hungry developing countries, such as Nigeria, Tanzania, Uganda, India, and Iraq, the number of cases found has varied from one per 1,000 to 1 per cent of the people examined. This difference is quite astonishing.

The cause of hiatus hernia seems to be the same as that which leads to haemorrhoids. A low-fibre, high-sugar diet leads to constipation and to straining when trying to open the constipated bowel. It has been estimated that straining to evacuate a constipated bowel puts the pressure inside the abdominal cavity up to very high levels. The unnaturally high pressure may be an important cause of hiatus hernia. And in Britain, where women tend to be more constipated than men, the higher frequency of the disease among women could be explained by this observation.

The prevention and possible treatment of the disease is to make sure that the diet contains sufficient fibre, and, if it doesn't, to add bran to the diet, and to make sure that the bowel is opened regularly.

Three other intestinal disorders have been related to a lack of fibre in our diet. These are appendicitis, irritable bowel syndrome, and diverticular disease. At present there is insufficient information to determine the protective role of fibre, if there is any, in their prevention, although some gastro-enterologists believe that the symptoms of diverticular disease are reduced if the diet contains increased amounts of dietary fibre.

Coronary Heart Disease

There is evidence that a diet that contains about twice the amount of fibre as the average Western diet reduces the chance of coronary heart disease by helping to lower the cholesterol in the blood. This is an important health issue and is discussed in Chapter 10.

Non-starch polysaccharide, or dietary fibre, is one of the components of complex carbohydrates, along with starch. These components are beneficial to health, and more foods that are rich in complex carbohydrates should be eaten. These foods are cereals, vegetables, legumes, tubers, and fruits.

It is probable that the daily intake of dietary fibre should be increased from the current 20 g to at least 30 g.

The fibre is best obtained from food, but some people may chose to eat oat or rice bran, which contains fibre. The

Good Sources of Fibre (over 3.5 g per 100 g of food)

	g		g
Wholemeal bread	8.5	per slice	2.5
White bread	3.5	per slice	1.0
White pasta		per serving	2.5
Brown pasta			5.0
All Bran	26.7	per serving	9.5
Cornflakes	11.0		3.0
Puffed Wheat	15.4		5.0
Grape Nuts	7.0		2.5
Muesli	24.0		8.0
Porridge	11.0		5.0
Weetabix	12.7		4.0
Crispbread	11.7		3.0
Digestive biscuits	5.5		1.5
Baked beans	18.3		9.0
Broccoli	3.6		3.6
Brussels sprouts	4.2		4.2
Peas	6.0		6.0
Spinach	4.5		4.5
Sweetcorn	4.5		4.5
Yam	4.0		4.0
Apricots (dried)	24.0		
Currants (black, red)	8.5	per ½ punnet	9.0
Figs (dried)	18.5		
Passion fruit	15.9		
Prunes	16.1		
Raisins	6.8		
Raspberries	7.5	per ½ punnet	7.5
Sultanas	7.0		
Nuts	9.5	per 30 g	3.0

Source: McCance and Widdowson, **Composition of Foods**.

Aim to eat 30–40 g of dietary fibre most days. If you choose to eat oat or rice bran limit it to 1 tablespoonful a day, which will provide 14 g a day. More than this may interfere with the absorption of calcium, iron, and zinc.

amount of oat or rice bran eaten should be limited to no more than 14 g a day, as too much dietary fibre, unless eaten in a diet rich in complex carbohydrates may cause problems.

When dietary fibre is increased, especially if you choose to eat bran or one of the over-the-counter preparations found in pharmacies, you will often notice that you develop flatulence, and pass more wind, often to your embarrassment. The production of wind is due to the action of bacteria on the largely insoluble fibre component of dietary fibre in the large bowel. The bacteria cause the fibre to ferment. After a while your body becomes used to the extra fibre and the problem ceases.

The message is if you decide to increase your dietary fibre, and particularly if you add fibre to your diet, rather than eating more complex carbohydrates, to help treat or prevent constipation and varicose veins, or to help prevent bowel cancer and coronary heart disease, change your diet slowly. You won't change the bowel habits of a lifetime overnight. The belching, abdominal distension, and excessive passing of wind will eventually go, so persist!

A potentially more serious problem is the eating of large quantities of wholemeal cereal or brown rice instead of more complex carbohydrates in a balanced diet. This is because wholemeal cereal and brown rice contain quantities of a substance called phytate as well as fibre. Phytate and fibre interfere with the absorption of calcium, iron, and zinc from the gut by combining with these minerals. The degree of interference is related to individual sensitivity, but it does constitute a problem when the bulk of the diet is made of wholemeal cereal. In childhood, calcium deficiency may cause rickets, and in adults it may cause osteomalacia. A deficiency of zinc may be a factor in the reduced height and the poor development of the sexual organs, which is fairly common in some west Asian countries.

The average diet of people in developed countries provides enough extra calcium in dairy foods, such as milk and cheese, and sufficient zinc in protein-rich foods such as meat, to counteract the effects of phytate, should wholemeal cereal be eaten. But when a balanced diet is not eaten, reliance on wholemeal bread, unless calcium, iron, and zinc have been added, may lead to malnutrition and the appearance of disease.

A balanced view and a balanced diet are needed.

9 ALCOHOL—FOR YOUR STOMACH'S SAKE?

● ●

From the time that the nomadic hunter–gatherers settled down and began farming, it was observed that grain would ferment to make a brew which, if drunk, produced pleasant effects. Today alcohol continues to produce the pleasant effects, and plays an important role in our social and ritual life, all over the world except in Islamic countries.

Alcohol is produced from the fermention of carbohydrates contained in cereals, fruits, vegetables, and sugar. The fermentation is due to the action of yeast on the carbohydrate. When alcohol is imbibed, it rapidly reaches the stomach and, because it is highly soluble in water, it is rapidly absorbed through the wall of the stomach to enter the blood. If the stomach is empty, the absorption is very rapid; if there is food in the stomach, the rate of absorption is a little slower, as the food–alcohol mix passes into the small intestine. If the alcoholic beverage is carbonated (as in sparkling wine, or when soda water, ginger ale, or tonic water is added to a drink), the rate of absorption through the walls of the stomach is increased.

The alcohol from the beverage enters the bloodstream, and its peak blood concentration is reached in twenty minutes or a bit longer if food is eaten at the same time as the drink is imbibed. It is carried to the liver, where it is broken down by enzymes, and distributed to all parts of the body, the amount of alcohol in a tissue being proportionate to the water content of the tissue. Over the period of an hour after imbibing an alcoholic beverage, about 10 g of the contained alcohol is broken down into carbon dioxide, releasing energy.

Repeated excessive drinking will in the long term affect these organs and tissues

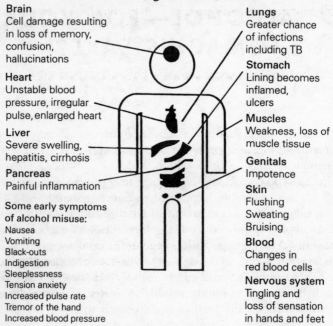

Brain
Cell damage resulting in loss of memory, confusion, hallucinations

Heart
Unstable blood pressure, irregular pulse, enlarged heart

Liver
Severe swelling, hepatitis, cirrhosis

Pancreas
Painful inflammation

Some early symptoms of alcohol misuse:
Nausea
Vomiting
Black-outs
Indigestion
Sleeplessness
Tension anxiety
Increased pulse rate
Tremor of the hand
Increased blood pressure

Lungs
Greater chance of infections including TB

Stomach
Lining becomes inflamed, ulcers

Muscles
Weakness, loss of muscle tissue

Genitals
Impotence

Skin
Flushing
Sweating
Bruising

Blood
Changes in red blood cells

Nervous system
Tingling and loss of sensation in hands and feet

FIG. 9.1. *The effect of alcohol on the body*

The more alcohol that is imbibed over a short period of time, the higher the blood concentration becomes, and the longer it takes for the alcohol to be broken down. In addition, it appears that the rate of conversion to carbon dioxide depends on many factors: the body build (lean people are more efficient at metabolizing alcohol than fat people), age, inheritance (there is possibly a gene for sensitivity to alcohol), among others.

Alcohol is a sedative: it induces sleep. In the period before sedation, alcohol produces a feeling of well-being and relaxation. This mood-change may lead to a reduction of inhibi-

Myths about Alcohol

Myth	Fact
Alcohol stops you having a cold.	It has no effect on the progress of the virus, but may make you feel better because it is a sedative.
Black coffee helps you sober up.	Coffee does not increase the rate at which you metabolize alcohol, but it may counteract the sedative properties of alcohol.
Taking multivitamins stops hangovers.	It does not.
Alcohol increases sexual desire.	In small quantities alcohol reduces inhibitions; in larger quantities it promotes sleep, not sex.
Alcohol warms you up if you are cold.	Alcohol increases the body temperature for a short time, but after that it causes heat loss, as it dilates blood vessels in the skin.

tions, to animation and talkativeness. As the brain cells absorb alcohol, the performance of the person is affected, particularly if co-ordination and judgement is required, as in driving a motor vehicle. Aggressiveness may also occur, but the next day the person will remember little of what happened.

As the concentration of alcohol in the blood and the body tissues rises, the sedative properties of alcohol become more apparent. Slurring of speech, nausea, and a desire to sleep replace talkativeness or aggression.

People who become addicted to alcohol, chronic alcoholics, often eat very little food, partly because the alcohol causes gastritis, which destroys their appetite, partly because of the high energy content of alcohol, and partly because they spend most of their available money on alcoholic beverages. As a result they frequently develop nutritional deficiencies, particularly of the vitamin B group. Deficiency in thiamin results in damage to the brain, including the death of many brain cells. This causes mental confusion, staggering gait, and visual disturbance (Wernicke's encephalopathy). The condition responds to injections of thiamin if treated early enough.

In severe cases, the person loses his or her memory and is unable to acquire new knowledge, a condition called Korsakoff's psychosis. Thiamin is not so successful in treating people with Korsakoff's psychosis; over three-quarters remain mentally damaged permanently.

Hangovers

If sufficient alcohol has been drunk, a hangover may result. The symptoms of nausea, dryness of the mouth, headache, dizziness, and over-sensitivity to noise and light occur as the body metabolizes the alcohol. The nausea is due to the irritating effect of alcohol on the stomach and on a centre in the brain. The headache is due to dilatation of blood vessels in the brain, and, in some people, to a sensitivity to substances called amines in the beverage (for example, red wine made from Shiraz grapes is often blamed). The dryness is due to dehydration, because alcohol affects kidney hormones, which regulate the loss of water from the body.

Alcohol as a source of energy

As mentioned, alcohol releases energy when it is broken down in the body, and this energy adds to the body's energy intake. The alcoholic content of different drinks varies as does the energy released.

The Benefits of Alcohol

Alcohol helps people to relax and adds to pleasant social intercourse by reducing inhibitions. In small quantities (no

Standard drinks (one unit)	Energy content (kJ)
285 ml (10 oz.) ordinary beer	500
570 ml (20 oz.) of light beer	380
120 ml (4 oz. or one glass) of red or white wine	350
60 ml (2 oz.) of sherry or port	350
30 ml (1 oz., a pub measure) of spirits	290

A safe level of alcohol consumption is, for men, no more than 30 units a week, and for women, no more than 15 units a week.

more than two 'standard drinks' a day) alcohol may reduce the risk of a heart attack. But too much alcohol makes it a health hazard.

The Dangers of Alcohol

In most Western countries, about 10 per cent of all adults in the population have health problems due to alcohol. A number of these people are alcohol-addicted—they have the alcohol-dependence syndrome. They have a compulsion to drink, and a steady, stereotypical pattern of drinking at regular, predictable intervals. Drinking is for them the most important thing they do, taking primacy over everything else; they have repeated withdrawal symptoms (the 'shakes', agitation, nausea, or hallucinations), which can be relieved by drinking. People with an alcoholic dependence are usually in their forties, but increasingly the syndrome is occurring among younger people, and some elderly people are affected for the first time.

Alcohol-related illness causes considerable social and economic problems. It has been estimated in the USA that one person in twenty-five who works in industry or commerce has an alcohol problem.

Alcohol is a factor in over 40 per cent of road crashes, and is a cause of many cases of domestic (and other) violence.

Even if no more than five standard drinks are taken each

day, alcohol damages the brain, killing brain cells and shrinking the brain. The damage to the brain is more likely to occur if the person frequently goes on drinking bouts.

If a person drinks heavily for a number of years, and particularly if he or she has a genetic sensitivity to alcohol, the alcohol may cause liver damage. This shows at first as an enlargement of the liver, but over a period of time, as more liver cells are damaged, the liver shrinks, becomes hard, and ceases to function properly.

Alcohol is associated with a tendency to high blood pressure, and may be involved in cancers of the gastro-intestinal tract, particularly the oesophagus.

Given all these adverse effects, it is perhaps surprising that some people continue to drink alcohol in excess. But they do so for the relaxation it produces and because it is an accepted social activity.

In addition, alcohol adds to the chance that you will become fat. For example, if you drink four cans of beer a day you will increase your energy intake by 2,000 kJ a day, the equivalent of 6 g of fat. Over a year this may add about 2 kg to your

....

Are You a Sensible Drinker?

Do you find it difficult to refuse alcohol?	*Yes*	(B)	*No*	(A)
Can you enjoy a day without alcohol?	*Yes*	(A)	*No*	(B)
Do you know how much alcohol you drink each week?	*Yes*	(A)	*No*	(B)
Do you drink alcohol before driving?	*Yes*	(B)	*No*	(A)
Is alcohol spoiling your sport?	*Yes*	(B)	*No*	(A)
Have your family or any of your friends ever made comments against your drinking?	*Yes*	(B)	*No*	(A)
Do you drink within 'sensible' limits?	*Yes*	(A)	*No*	(B)

If you scored 0 to 2 Bs, you are a sensible drinker; if you had 3 to 4 Bs, take care, and try to make a few changes; and if you had 5 to 7 Bs, you are heading for a drinking problem.

....

weight if you continue to eat your usual diet. Many drinkers do not eat much food, so the increase in weight will be less, but nevertheless it will slowly build up. If you have a pre-dinner whisky, and drink half a bottle of wine with dinner every day for a year, you will add 1 kg to your weight each year.

10 THE FATS OF DEATH?

• •

When we talk about fats, we think of butter, margarine, cooking fat or oil, and the fat we can see on the meat we buy. We do not usually think about the fat that we do not see. But fat is hidden in many manufactured foods, ranging from nearly 40 per cent of the weight of the food in many cheeses, potato crisps, and chocolate, to a mere trace in most vegetables and fruits. Hidden fat is also contained in cakes, biscuits, puddings, and sauces. This is the problem with fats: most people do not know how much of it they are eating.

Fats have value: they provide a concentrated source of energy, but unless you are an Eskimo they are indigestible in quantity. Fats improve the taste of food, and in the diet that Western people choose to eat, they provide nearly 40 per cent of the daily energy intake. This amount can cause health problems, particularly heart disease.

Nutritionists recommend that we should reduce the amount of fats in our diet to provide no more than than 30 per cent of our energy needs.

What is the basis for this recommendation? What we call fats are called lipids by nutritionists. Lipids are formed from fatty acids linked with other substances. The fatty acids that make up the lipids may be saturated, polyunsaturated, or mono-unsaturated, and the proportion of each in the diet plays a role in the development of heart disease.

Most saturated fats are 'bad' fats (because they raise the level of cholesterol in the blood), polyunsaturated fats are 'good' fats (provided not too much of them is eaten), and most mono-unsaturated fats are also 'good' fats.

Saturated fats are mainly animal fats (including dairy products). Only two vegetable fats are saturated: these are palm and coconut oil, which is used as a base for ice-cream manufacture. The greatest proportion of saturated fats that we eat comes not from meat or milk, but from the hidden fats in the fatty processed meats—sausages, bacon, and salami—and in cakes, biscuits, pastries, chocolates, and cheeses. Most nutritionists consider that we eat too much saturated fat, which tends to raise the level of cholesterol in the blood.

Saturated fats currently provide about 35 per cent of our energy needs. Nutritionists suggest that for better health we should reduce the energy provided by saturated fats to less than 20 per cent.

Polyunsaturated fats are usually vegetable in origin but are also found in a wide variety of foods including fish, crustaceans, and game. There are several kinds of poly-unsaturated fat. In vegetable oils, omega-6 fatty acids predominate. In fish, particularly cold-water fish, omega-3 fatty acids predominate.

In Western countries polyunsaturated fats provide about 7 per cent of energy intake, and could be safely increased to provide about 10 per cent of our daily energy needs.

Mono-unsaturated fats, which are found in olive oil, peanut oil, peanuts, and avocados are beneficial to health. People living in Mediterranean countries eat more mono-unsaturated fats than other Europeans and have less coronary heart disease. However, they eat less total fats, as well, and this may be an additional reason for the lower incidence of heart disease. Mono-unsaturated fats act like polyunsaturated fats in protecting against heart attack. Mono-unsaturated fats lower the 'bad' cholesterol, low-density lipoprotein (LDL), as much as polyunsaturated fats do. Most people living in Australia, Britain, or the USA derive few kilojoules from this kind of fat, unless we eat a Mediterranean-type diet. As we shall see, there are health benefits in eating such a diet.

Although fats still contribute about 40 per cent of our energy needs, in the past twenty years there has been a decline in the proportion of saturated fats eaten and an increase in the amount of polyunsaturated fats. This change has coincided with a falling incidence of coronary heart disease. A reason may be, as dietary experiments have shown, that replacing saturated fats with polyunsaturated and mono-unsaturated fats, even without reducing the total contribution of fats to the diet, leads to a fall in plasma cholesterol.

The theory that diets which provide a large quantity of fat, particularly cholesterol-raising saturated fats, and in consequence cholesterol, are a factor in causing heart disease was based originally on the observation that the incidence of coronary heart disease differed widely between countries. In 1985, according to the World Health Organization, the five countries with the highest death rate of middle-aged men (aged 45 to 69) in 1985 were Finland, Scotland, England and Wales, Australia, and the USA. The four countries with the lowest death rate from heart disease among middle-aged men in 1985 were Japan, France, Italy, and Poland.

What accounts for this difference? Investigations have shown that a majority of the people of the countries that have the highest death rates from heart disease eat a diet that contains far more saturated fat than the majority of the people in countries that have the lowest death rates from heart disease. For example, most people in Australia, Britain, and the USA obtain over one-third of their daily energy intake from dairy products and meat, while most people in Japan obtain only 4 per cent of their energy intake from dairy products and meat, and twice as much of their energy needs as Americans from cereal grains, vegetables, legumes, and fruits. The saturated fat content of the diet of most Italians falls in between that of the Americans and the Japanese.

Within countries such as England and Wales, Australia, and the USA, the lower the social class of the man (and to a lesser extent the woman) the greater is the chance of having a heart attack. This is, in part, due to dietary habits, as poorer people have less choice of foods and tend to buy fatty foods, but other factors are also involved.

Evidence is now available which clearly incriminates the amount of total fat, and particularly saturated fat, which provides cholesterol, in the diet as a risk factor in heart disease.

Today there is widespread agreement among cardiologists that saturated fats in the diet are intimately involved in the development of coronary heart disease. There is also agreement that the higher the level of cholesterol in the blood, the greater is the chance that heart disease will develop. This does not mean, however, that a high blood cholesterol is the cause of coronary heart disease, as many people with a high blood cholesterol have no evidence of atherosclerosis, and the blood cholesterol level of many people who have a heart attack is in the normal range.

How Heart Disease Occurs

Inevitably we all die. The two most common causes of death are heart disease and cancer. Deaths from heart disease are most common after the age of 69, and are twice as common in men as in women. But deaths from heart disease also occur before the age of 69, at a time when a person could be said to be in the prime of life, usually when he or she is working, so that the death reduces the family income considerably. Loss of income is only one result of premature death: the loss of one's partner in a relationship may have a devastating effect on the emotional and often the physical life of the surviving partner.

For these reasons, in recent years much community and professional concern has been expressed about heart disease as a cause of premature death. Since the late 1970s the death rate from heart disease has been falling, but numbers of apparently healthy middle-aged men and women still die from heart disease.

Can any preventive measures be taken to reduce the

numbers? To answer this question it is useful to understand how coronary heart disease and heart attacks occur.

How Heart Attacks Occur

A heart attack is due to the blocking of one or more of the main arteries, the coronary arteries, which supply the heart muscle. The block is due to a process called *atherosclerosis*. Atherosclerosis comes from two Greek words *athere* and *sclerosis*: *athere* means mush or porridge and *sclerosis* means narrowing. This is what happens to the arteries.

Atherosclerosis of the arteries, particularly the main artery, the aorta, and the coronary arteries, may begin very early in life and progress slowly over the years, or regress if corrective action is taken. Just how long it takes is uncertain.

Fatty streaks have been found in the arteries of teenagers; they are more common in people in their twenties. For example, autopsies on soldiers killed in Korea and Vietnam, and of victims of violence in the USA, have shown that over 10 per cent of healthy young men under the age of 30 had signs of atherosclerosis in their arteries. If the young man had smoked, the chance of finding evidence of atherosclerosis doubled.

If the disease progresses, the fatty streaks increase in size, and by the time the person has reached his or her thirties they will have become patches, called plaques, in the arteries. In one autopsy study of men aged 30 to 34, 15 per cent had evidence of plaque formation, and in smokers the rate was double at 30 per cent. In contrast, autopsies of 373 Ugandans aged 60 and over, carried out by Dr Drury in 1972, showed that only 1.6 per cent of them had evidence of atherosclerotic plaques in their arteries. This suggests that there may be something that people living in developed countries do (or don't do) or eat that increases the chance of atherosclerosis.

The plaques are usually circular in shape, have a roughened surface, and bulge to a greater or lesser degree into the cavity of the artery. They are filled with foamy cells, which are full of cholesterol.

Cholesterol is made in the body and is a constituent of all cell membranes. It is also a starting substance for the synthesis of many important hormones. In this respect it is a vital substance. As well as being made in the body, cholesterol is ingested into the body in foods rich in saturated fat, together with another fatty substance, triglyceride.

Cholesterol and triglycerides from food are absorbed through the wall of the intestines and are taken into the bloodstream where they are attached, for transport, to substances called lipoproteins. Four classes of lipoprotein have been described, which depend on the size of the particle of lipoprotein. The four kinds of lipoprotein have different transport functions.

The largest lipoprotein is the chylomicron, which transports most of the triglycerides and some of the cholesterol from the intestines to the liver. Next comes the very-low-density lipoprotein (VLDL) which carries some triglycerides and some cholesterol. Then comes low-density lipoprotein (LDL), which mainly carries cholesterol from the liver to the peripheral tissues. Finally, there is the smallest-sized lipoprotein, high-density lipoprotein (HDL). Its main function is to get rid of excess cholesterol in the tissues by transporting it back to the liver, where it is broken down and excreted.

Triglycerides are broken down in the body into fatty acids, releasing energy, so that they cause little problem except by adding to the energy intake. The effects of extra cholesterol on health is different. If there is an excess of cholesterol in the diet, or if you have inherited an abnormality of lipid transport, the extra cholesterol is deposited in the tissues, particularly in the cells that line the inner surface (the lumen) of the arteries. Here it becomes 'rancid', and the rancid cholesterol attacts blood cells called monocytes, which attach themselves to the cholesterol and engulf it, creating foamy cells. At first these cells form fatty streaks under the cells lining the inner surface of the blood vessel. As time passes, if excess cholesterol continues to be available, the foamy cells multiply, swell, and project into the lumen of

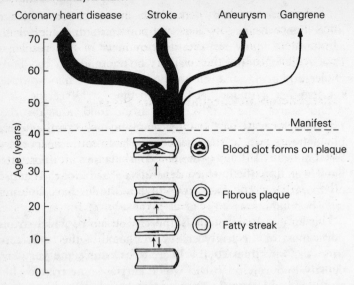

FIG. 10.1. *The development of atherosclerosis*

the artery, forming the plaque. As the blood pulses turbulently past the plaque, small blood cells, called platelets, attach to the roughened surface, and may start a blood clot, which over time may become hard, because calcium is deposited in it. If the plaque is in one of the coronary arteries, and if a blood clot forms on its surface, the artery will become progressively narrowed, reducing the blood flow to the part of the heart muscle it supplies. This may cause angina. Sometimes the blood flowing past the plaque is not reduced sufficiently to cause angina, but a clot may suddenly form on the surface of the plaque, blocking the entire lumen of the coronary artery. This prevents blood flowing to the part of the heart muscle supplied by the artery and, in consequence, the muscle fibres in the area supplied by the artery die. This causes severe, long-lasting chest pain, and sometimes sudden death. In other words, the person has a heart attack (Figure 10.1).

This brief, simplistic description shows the role cholesterol and its carriers, low-density lipoprotein and high-density lipoprotein, play in the development of atherosclerosis, particularly that of the coronary arteries.

Risk Factors in Coronary Heart Disease

Studies over the past twenty years have shown that certain behaviours add to the chance of a premature heart attack, that is before the age of 70. These risk factors are cumulative, and it is unrealistic to concentrate on one alone. At present the greatest emphasis is on reducing the level of cholesterol in the blood, for the reasons given above. Dietary fats and cholesterol as risk factors for heart disease have already been discussed. It is equally important that the other risk factors are discussed if heart attacks are to be reduced among people under 70.

Apart from dietary saturated fats and cholesterol, the other risk factors for coronary heart disease are:

- genetic
- cigarette-smoking
- high blood pressure
- lack of exercise—sloth
- obesity.

The Genetic Factor—Choosing the Right Parents

One family in every 250 has a genetic defect that makes some of its members produce an excess of lipoprotein, usually LDL, and consequently they have high blood levels of LDL cholesterol. (More accurately, they have few or no tissue receptors for LDL so that the lipid increases in their blood.) They develop small raised yellow patches containing cholesterol on various parts of their body, and particularly in their arteries. These plaques put them at considerable risk of a heart attack. Over half of all heart attacks in men under the age of 55 occur in these families. This risk is considerably reduced if the affected people take measures to reduce the level of LDL in their blood and tissues. This can be done by diet and exercise, but most people with this genetic disorder will require cholesterol-lowering drugs.

Members of other families, in which a close relative has had a heart attack at an early age, and whose blood lipid patterns are normal, also have an increased risk.

Cigarette-Smoking and Heart Disease

Three major investigations have shown that tobacco-smoking is a risk factor for heart disease. In an investigation of over 1 million men in the USA, two scientists, Drs Hammond and Garfinkle, found that men aged 40 to 49 who smoked had three times the risk of a heart attack. In England Sir Richard Doll and Dr Hill found that moderate cigarette-smoking trebled the risk of dying from coronary heart disease among men aged 45 to 54. The Framingham study in the USA, which has been going on for thirty-six years, has found that smokers have double the risk of a heart attack. In Australia, the National Heart Foundation has reported that a person aged between 45 and 54 who smokes 10 to 19 cigarettes a day has double the risk of a heart attack; and smoking more than 20 cigarettes a day trebles the risk.

That is the bad news. The good news is that if you give up smoking, your risk of dying from a heart attack falls steadily. After four years it is the same as that of someone who has never smoked.

High Blood Pressure and Coronary Heart Disease

Hypertension, or high blood pressure, is undoubtedly an accelerating factor in heart disease. For example, in 1976 Professor Morris recorded that among a group of middle-aged London bus drivers, who were studied for 10 years, the higher the initial blood pressure, the greater the risk of developing coronary heart disease. A 1990 analysis of all reported investigations confirmed these findings. In the USA a similar investigation showed the same result, and it also showed that by reducing the high blood pressure a substantial reduction in heart attacks, strokes, and heart failure was obtained. 'Now', writes Professor Morris, 'moderate and severe hypertension can be lowered by today's potent and fairly well tolerated medicines.' But of course, you can't reduce the blood pressure until you find those people in the community who have high blood pressure, and offer them treatment.

The test, as many people know, is really quite simple. In 1905 a Russian physician, Korotkoff, discovered that if a pressure cuff was applied to the upper arm, the blood pressure could be measured by pumping air into the cuff to obstruct the flow of blood through the main artery of the arm. The air was then released slowly, until the blood flowed again, and the sounds of the pulse (which reflects the heartbeat) were listened to over the artery in the fold of the elbow, using a stethoscope. With each heartbeat the blood pressure rises to a peak. This is called the systolic pressure. In between heartbeats the pressure falls to a lower level. This is called the diastolic pressure. By pumping up the cuff so that no blood flows through the artery and then releasing the air slowly, the blood flows in squirts and thumps loudly on the artery wall which the doctor can hear through the stethoscope. This is the systolic pressure. As the cuff empties, the character of the thumps changes and becomes soft. The blood pressure varies throughout the day and responds to all kinds of stress or emotion, when it tends to rise. During sleep it is at its lowest. The temporary rises are normal and natural, but the doctor tries to take a resting pressure.

High blood pressure—hypertension—is diagnosed when the blood pressure is constantly above a certain level. In adults this level is usually said to be 150 mm of mercury for the systolic pressure, and 95 mm of mercury for the diastolic pressure. About one person in ten over the age of 30 has a blood pressure above this level, and this individual is at increased risk of having a heart attack or a stroke when older. The risk is doubled if the diastolic blood pressure remains persistently above 110 mm of mercury. Not every person with high blood pressure needs drugs. For many, weight reduction, regular exercise, reduction of stress, and giving up smoking may be all that are needed. For others drugs will be required.

Lack of Exercise and Coronary Heart Disease

The benefit of regular enjoyable exercise tailored to the person's age and muscle-strength in reducing the risk of a heart attack has been conclusively established. People who do not take regular exercise are twice as likely to suffer a heart attack as those who do. Given this knowledge it is surprising that relatively few people take regular exercise. A study in Britain, in 1990, of adolescents aged 11 to 16 found that less than half took exercise three times a week. In the same year a study in the USA showed that 58 per cent of adult Americans led a sedentary life and did not take regular exercise.

The exercise need not be excessively strenuous, as was suggested some years ago. Physicians have found that the same benefit can be had from exercise such as walking briskly for thirty minutes three times a week, cycling regularly, or climbing five flights of stairs three times a week.

Obesity and Coronary Heart Disease

Whether obesity in itself is a contributor to heart disease has not been determined. However, obese people are more likely to have high blood pressure, eat diets rich in saturated fats, have a high blood level of cholesterol, smoke cigarettes, and, often, not take much exercise.

The long-term study of the citizens of the town of Framingham has shown that obese people have an increased risk of dying from coronary heart disease. The scientists agree that 'some but not all of the increased cardiovascular risk associated with obesity is attributed to the worsening of the risk factors', and add: 'Because of the influence of weight on the major cardiovascular risk factors, weight control is an important feature of a preventive program against cardiovascular disease.'

Reducing the Risk of Developing Coronary Heart Disease

All the risk factors mentioned above are involved in reducing the size of the coronary arteries, by plaque formation. The two risk factors receiving the most attention at present are a raised blood cholesterol, due, in most cases, to a diet that contains a high proportion of saturated fats; and sloth, the lack of regular physical exercise.

Determining the Blood Cholesterol Level

Three well-conducted investigations relating the blood cholesterol to the risk of a heart attack within ten years stand out among much research that has been carried out in the past two decades. These are the Framingham study, the Lipid Research Clinic Study (conducted in the USA), and the Helsinki Heart Study.

These studies demonstrate that the higher the blood cholesterol, the greater is the chance of a heart attack. The medical scientists who designed and conducted the investigations agree that if a person has several risk factors, the chance of coronary heart disease increases (see Figure 10.2), so it is important not to concentrate solely on reducing or eliminating only one of them. The studies show that if the level of blood cholesterol is reduced by 10 per cent, the risk of a heart attack is reduced by 20 per cent. As one person in four between the ages of 40 and 70 who has a heart attack dies soon after the attack, a considerable number of premature deaths could be prevented if strategies were adopted, one of which is to reduce the level of blood cholesterol by eating a sensible diet and by exercising regularly. (See page 92 for the other preventive strategies.)

These facts are generally accepted, but there is also controversy about blood cholesterol and its relation to coronary heart disease. The questions are: Should all men and women have their blood cholesterol level measured, and if so, at what age should the first test be made, and how often thereafter? What is the optimum range in which the blood cho-

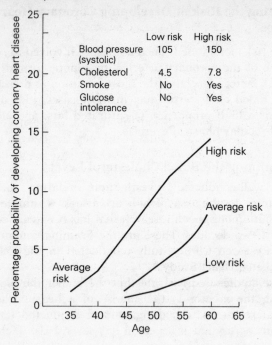

Source: Data from W. B. Kannel, T. R. Dawber, and
D. L. McGee, *Circulation*, 61(1980), 1179–82.

FIG. 10.2. *Probability of developing coronary heart disease in eight years according to age*

lesterol should lie to reduce the risk of a heart attack? If the blood cholesterol is high, how should it be treated and at what level should treatment with potent drugs be initiated?

Who should have their blood cholesterol measured?

In the Framingham study men whose blood cholesterol was measured when they were between the ages of 30 and 49 at the start of the study were followed for thirty-six years. During these years regular physical and laboratory investigations (including cholesterol measurements) were conducted. By then some of the men had developed coronary heart disease

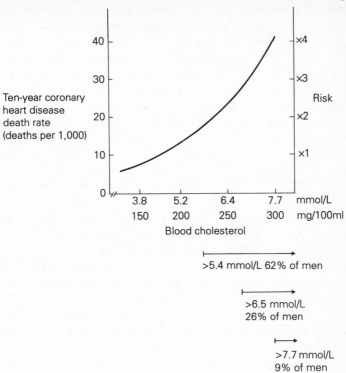

FIG. 10.3. *Risk of heart disease in relation to blood cholesterol level in men aged 30 to 64 (survey of 362,000 US men)*

and some had died. The scientists found that the men whose blood cholesterol was under 5.5 mmol per litre when aged 30 to 39 had a fairly small chance of dying from a heart attack over the next 30 years, while men whose blood cholesterol was higher than 6.5 mmol per litre when aged 30 to 39 had a much higher chance of having a heart attack during the period of the study.

The relationship between the blood cholesterol level and the risk of a heart attack was examined in a study of 362,000 American men aged 30 to 64 (see Figure 10.3). It will be noted that 62 per cent of the men had a blood cholesterol of more than 5.4 mmol per litre, and 62 per cent of the men had a blood cholesterol of more than 6.5 mmol per litre. The curve of the ten-year coronary heart disease death rate increased more rapidly for those whose level was over 5.5 mmol per litre. It would perhaps be a good idea to try to get your blood cholesterol below that level.

However, total blood cholesterol, which we have been discussing, is only one factor in the cholesterol story. The levels of the 'good' HDL cholesterol and the 'bad' LDL cholesterol are also important. This raises the question of whether and when HDL should be measured and LDL calculated. In the Framingham study, for example, it was found that an HDL level lower than 1.0 mmol per litre added considerably to the risk of a heart attack.

The present opinion, or at least that held by most physicians, is that HDL and LDL need be measured only if the person's total blood cholesterol is higher than 6.5 mmol per litre. Some physicians rely on the ratio of total cholesterol to HDL cholesterol, while others prefer to calculate the ratio of LDL to HDL, to make a prediction about the chance of the development of heart disease.

At present there is no consensus among physicians about which of the calculations provides the most accurate prediction about the risk of a heart attack.

At what age should blood cholesterol be first measured?

There is no consensus about this question either. If the age of 35 is chosen, when coronary heart disease is uncommon in men, and rare in women, the screening of the entire population would be costly and not without psychological risk. As mentioned, all that a raised level of cholesterol indicates is that the person is at greater risk of having a heart attack than a person whose blood cholesterol is 'normal'. It does not indicate that he or she will certainly have a heart attack at some time in the future. For example, in the USA over 60 million men are estimated to have a blood cholesterol above 5.5 mmol per litre, but only 1.5 million will have a heart attack.

A problem is that some people whose blood cholesterol is raised may become obsessional about their blood cholesterol and may resort to medication to reduce its level instead of reducing all the risk factors for coronary heart disease by eating a prudent diet, by taking exercise, and by ceasing to smoke.

If your blood cholesterol is high what action should you take?

The most logical way to reduce a high blood cholesterol is to change your diet so that you eat smaller quantities of foods that contain saturated fats. This does not mean that you must avoid all cholesterol-containing foods. There are several diets that enable you to reduce your intake of saturated fats without distorting your eating habits too badly. One such diet is shown on pages 164–5.

Many books are appearing that try to persuade you that you can reduce a high blood cholesterol easily, painlessly, and quickly. Some of them advise you to eat a low-fat diet, but most try to persuade you to rely mainly on eating quantities of oat bran or rice bran, to obtain a quick result. As was mentioned in Chapter 8, certain kinds of dietary fibre, taken in sufficient amounts, help to reduce blood cholesterol levels. There is now good evidence that bran obtained from oats, rice, and probably other sources have this effect. But their effect is less than the reduction achieved by eating a diet low in saturated fats. In fact, bran alone reduces the level of blood cholesterol by only 5 per cent at the most.

Eating a diet low in saturated fats and adding bran if you wish is not enough. You should also take regular enjoyable exercise.

When should drugs be taken to reduce the blood cholesterol level?

Most physicians agree that if a raised blood cholesterol level is found on two or more examinations, with certain exceptions, you should first try to reduce the level by changing your diet, and by taking regular exercise. In some instances

How to Reduce the Chance of a Heart Attack

Diet
- Eat more vegetables and fruit.
- Eat more fish and more poultry, but do not eat the skin of the poultry as it contains a good deal of saturated fat.
- Eat lean meat rather than fatty, marbled meat.
- Grill the fish, poultry, and meat.
- Do not eat more than five eggs a week.
- Replace butter with polyunsaturated margarine, and spread it thinly! Choose a soft margarine with a high content ratio of polyunsaturated to saturated fat, as shown on the ingredients label.
- Eat more complex cereals (bread, preferably wholemeal), pasta, rice, oatmeal, and low-fat and low-sugar breakfast cereals.
- Eat few or no cakes, pasties, chocolate, and biscuits.
- Eat cream and ice-cream sparingly.
- Eat less sugar.
- Use mono-unsaturated oils (olive oil) or polyunsaturated fats for cooking when you have to use cooking oil at all.

Exercise
- Take more enjoyable exercise, and take it regularly.

Smoking
- If you smoke tobacco, stop.

Obesity
- If you are obese, try to reduce your weight.

Blood pressure
- Have your blood pressure measured each year after you reach the age of 30. If it is raised, consult your doctor for advice on ways to reduce it.

diet and exercise will reduce the blood cholesterol level by 20 to 25 per cent, but most people achieve only a 10 to 15 per cent reduction. If the diet and exercise regimen fails to reduce the blood cholesterol level over a period of about six months, and if the level is higher than 7.7 mmol per litre, drug treatment may be tried. The first drugs developed worked by binding the cholesterol in the food in the gut and so preventing it from being absorbed. They produced some rather unpleasant symptoms, mainly nausea, flatulence, and constipation, but were moderately effective in reducing the level of cholesterol in the blood. More recently a new type of drug has been developed which inhibits the action a liver enzyme, which is required for cholesterol to be synthesized and processed. These drugs produce a greater reduction in the level of cholesterol in the blood, are better tolerated, and produce fewer gastric upsets. In several multicentre studies the drugs have been found to reduce the blood cholesterol level by 25 per cent or more. It should be added that among people aged 40 to 59 who take these cholesterol-reducing drugs, their chance of *avoiding* a heart attack in any year is increased by only 1.7 per cent. Instead of an annual risk that 12 people in every 100 with very high blood cholesterol will have a heart attack, the risk is reduced to about 10 if they take the drugs.

11 THE VITAMIN CRAZE

• •

> Probably no single class of drugs has been the target of
> as much quackery, misunderstanding, misrepresenta-
> tion, and misuse as the vitamins, despite the fact that
> far more is known about these compounds, including
> their mechanism of action, than about any other group
> of substances in the United States Pharmacopoea.
>
> Paul Greengard, Professor of Pharmacology,
> Yale University School of Medicine

Everyone knows about vitamins. Unless enough of them are
provided in your diet you are likely to become ill because of
vitamin deficiency. What is less well known is that if you
ingest too much of certain vitamins you can become ill.

Technically, vitamins are organic compounds which are
involved in enzyme systems in the body and have to be
supplied in the diet, because the body has lost the ability
to make them. They were unknown until 1905, although
some perceptive nutritional scientists were beginning to
realize that food consisted of more than carbohydrates, fats,
and protein, and that other factors in the diet might be
responsible for protection against disease.

In 1912 a famous experiment was carried out by Frederick
Gowland Hopkins at the University of Cambridge. In an
attempt to discover the effects of diet on the growth of young
rats, he fed one group of rats a special diet consisting of
protein, fats, and carbohydrates, together with minerals. The
second group were given the same diet, but, in addition, each
rat was given about a teaspoonful of milk each day. The rats
given the special diet failed to grow, but those that received
the diet with the milk supplement thrived and developed

normally. After eighteen days Professor Hopkins withdrew the milk from the second group of rats and gave it to the first group. The results were the reverse of the first part of the experiment. The rats that had previously been deprived of milk now began to grow normally, while those that had previously had milk, but were now deprived of it, ceased to grow. Hopkins argued that milk contained an 'accessory factor' essential for growth. Because of his interest in proteins, which are made up of building-blocks of twenty amino acids, he believed that the accessory factor was an amino acid or an amine. Hopkins's paper was read by a Polish biochemist, Dr C. Funk, who called the new substances 'vitamines' because he thought that all the accessory factors were 'vital' amines. It is now known that most are not, but the name, without the final *e*, has stuck.

They were called vital amines, as they were found to be a vital portion of the enzymes, which help to carry out the body's functions, particularly processing the protein, the fat, and the carbohydrate from the food we eat.

Further research in several laboratories quickly identified other vital amines which, as they were discovered, were given a letter and called vitamins A, B, C, D, and E. In the past fifty years most of the vitamins have been identified chemically and given new chemical names, but the old alphabetical list persists, and is convenient.

Research has shown that the vitamins can be divided into two main groups: those that are soluble in fat and those that are soluble in water. The human body is unable to maintain a large store of the water-soluble vitamins B and C, and so deficiency disease is likely to arise after a few weeks or months if the diet is deficient in these vitamins. In contrast, the human liver stores the fat-soluble vitamins A, D, and E, so a well-fed adult has sufficient stores to protect him or her for months should the diet contain insufficient fat-soluble vitamins.

In the poor countries of the developing world, vitamin deficiency is not uncommon and causes much suffering. In

Western countries vitamin deficiency is rare. Most mothers eat enough good food to make sure that their foetus receives all the needed vitamins, and many pregnant women are given vitamin and iron supplements by their doctor. After birth most infants are either breast-fed, and their mother's milk provides the vitamins, or are given breast-milk substitutes, which have added vitamins. After weaning, most infants eat vitamin-containing foods, and so there is no problem. Most children, adolescents, and adults who eat a diet that includes bread and cereals, vegetables and fruit, meat or meat supplements, and dairy products obtain all the vitamins that they need for health and do not require vitamin supplements.

A few people in special circumstances are at risk of a vitamin deficiency and would benefit from vitamin supplements.

- Some premature babies may need vitamin E to reduce the risk of eye (retinal) damage caused by oxygen, although this is disputed.
- Newborn infants may need vitamin K_1, to prevent possible haemorrhage.
- Vegans, and especially their infants, need vitamin B_{12} supplements.
- Some women and children who live in northern Europe may require vitamin D in winter, as may children who have measles.
- A few elderly people and many chronic alcoholics eat a diet lacking in fruit and vegetables, and may need vitamin C.

Apart from these small groups of people, healthy people eating a healthy diet do not need vitamin supplements.

However, we are only too ready to believe the claims of skilful advertising that for 'perfect' health we need vitamin supplements. A study carried out in Australia, in 1984, of 1,000 people selected at random found that more than 50 per cent of the women and just under 40 per cent of the men took vitamins in addition to their regular diet. In the USA,

Britain, and Australia, at least US$20 (or its equivalent) is spent on vitamins each year for every man, woman, and child living in the country. That is a huge sum of money. Those who are most likely to purchase vitamin supplements are people who eat a good diet and are least in need of extra vitamins.

In this chapter we will look at the various vitamins and try to determine who may need vitamin supplements, and to dispel some of the myths about vitamins.

A Little Night-Blindness: Vitamin A, or Retinol

It was said that during the Second World War night fighter pilots were given additional rations of carrots (which contain vitamin A) so that they could see the enemy bombers better. The explanation was false, but it is true that deficiency in vitamin A leads to difficulty in vision when the light is dim.

Perhaps more important, at least to the millions of children in the hungry developing world, is that vitamin A is necessary for the growth of bone and for the normal growth and shedding of surface tissues. Every day the outermost cells of the skin, the gut, and the cornea of the eye die and are shed like leaves from a tree. But unlike the leaves on a tree, new cells immediately replace them. The process of shedding proceeds normally only if there is sufficient vitamin A circulating in the blood and seeping into the tissues. In the absence of an adequate supply, the surface tissues, particularly of the eyes, fail to shed the dead cells. These then collect on the surface and become dry and thickened. In the eyes a hazy opaque film across the cornea develops, and if it is not treated promptly by giving vitamin A, the cornea may soften and collapse, causing blindness.

Each year tens of thousands of children in the developing nations become permanently blind because of the lack of minute amounts of vitamin A in their daily food. Vitamin A is found mainly in butter, cheese, and milk and in liver and fish-liver oils. The body is also able to make it from the substance beta-carotene. This yellow pigment is found in green and yellow vegetables and fruits. In the body carotene is converted into vitamin A by the cells that line the gut.

In most tropical countries dairy foods are expensive, fish-liver oils and liver not eaten, and because of food taboos children can eat only certain fruits. In these areas diarrhoeal diseases are also common, and so less of the scarce vitamin A is absorbed at a time when more is needed.

The blindness due to vitamin A deficiency is rare in prosperous communities, but is still a cause of misery and despair in many developing nations. It has been calculated that in some areas, one in every hundred children under the age of 5 becomes blind as a result of vitamin A deficiency. This blindness is entirely preventable. If all the children were given supplements of vitamin A from birth, and if mothers learned about nutrition at school and in community centres, it would cease to be a problem. Vitamin A, or retinol, is cheap, and if sugar or salt used by people in the affected parts of the developing world were fortified with vitamin A, the blindness would disappear. It would cost no more than US 15 cents per head a year to eliminate this misery. To obtain the same amount of vitamin A needed from vegetables or fruit it would be necessary to eat three times as much of the former and twice as much of the latter.

Vitamin A, or more likely the beta-carotenes, may be valuable in preventing some health problems. For example, a study in the USA has found that a diet rich in beta-carotenes may retard the development of cardiovascular disease in people who show evidence of it. According to a study at Harvard University, men who had cardiovascular disease and who ate a diet rich in beta-carotenes had only half as many incidents of heart attacks, stroke, or sudden cardiac death compared with a control group of men who did not eat carotene-containing foods. The scientists say that the results are preliminary, and more research is needed before they can confirm the benefit of beta-carotenes in warding off cardiovascular disease.

Vitamin A or beta-carotenes may also be beneficial in preventing or changing the course of some cancers. Recent research found that in laboratory animals, vitamin A supplements in large doses, which are above the toxic level of the vitamin in humans, suppressed artificially induced cancer. This persuaded scientists in California to begin a study on human subjects to find out if supplementary capsules of vitamin A have the same effect. There are considerable problems with the study. First, it is not known whether vitamin A or carotenoids (substances related to carotene, found in vegetables) is the protective factor against cancer, if indeed it is protective. Second, there is concern that vitamin A in high doses may cause liver damage, so caution has to be exercised.

Until more information about the supposed benefit of vitamin A is available, it would be sensible for cancer sufferers to eat more carotene-rich foods, such as dark-green and deep-yellow vegetables and fruits, rather than taking vitamin A capsules in large doses.

Most people who live in the developed countries would be wise to eat more foods that contain beta-carotene. Vitamin A supplements are not necessary.

You should avoid taking large doses of vitamin A in high-dose capsules, as this may cause liver damage, if taken for a

....

Good Sources of Vitamin A and Carotene (Estimated daily requirement: 100 µg (retinol equivalent))

Vitamin A (pre-formed)	Carotene	
	Vegetables	*Fruits*
Liver	Broccoli	Apricots
Fish-liver oil	Carrots	Mangoes
Kidney	Kumera	Peaches
Milk (not low-fat)	Lettuce	Rock-melon
Butter	Pumpkin	
Cheese	Spinach	
Eggs		
Margarine (added)		

....

number of months. Another danger of high doses of vitamin A is the risk of birth defects. Women who are, or who may become pregnant, will get all the vitamin A they need from food, and should not eat liver or take any dietary supplements of vitamin A, including tablets and fish oils, except on the advice of a doctor, as the extra vitamin A increases the risk of the child having a birth defect.

The Case of the Twisted Bones (Vitamin D, or Cholecalciferol)

The Industrial Revolution of the nineteenth century in northwest Europe led to a drift of people from the rural areas to the new towns that had sprung up around the factories. As the revolution gathered momentum, the drift increased and the 'dark satanic mills', so graphically described by William Blake, were surrounded by small back-to-back workmen's cottages. The factories belched out smoke to cloud the sky so that even in summer the towns lay under the shroud of industrial pollution. Charles Dickens, writing in 1854, described one of these industrial towns in his book *Hard Times*, calling it Coketown:

It was a town of red brick, or of brick that would have been red if the smoke and ashes had allowed it; but, as matters stood it was a town of unnatural red and black like the painted face of a savage. It was a town of machinery and tall chimneys, out of which interminable serpents of smoke trailed themselves for ever and ever, and never got uncoiled.

Even in midsummer the sun was hidden:

Seen from a distance in such weather, Coketown lay shrouded in a haze of its own, which appeared impervious to the sun's rays. You only knew the town was there, because you knew there could have been no such sulky blotch upon the prospect without a town.

And within the town conditions were ideal for diseases to afflict the children of the workers:

In the hardest working part of Coketown, in the innermost fortifications of that ugly citadel where Nature was so strongly bricked out as killing airs and gases were bricked in; at the heart of the labyrinth of narrow courts upon courts and close streets upon streets . . . were built in an immense variety of stunted and crooked shapes as though every house put out a sign of the kind of people who might be expected to be born in it; lived the people.

The hours of work were long, the pay poor, and the threat of dismissal great. Food was indeed more plentiful than in rural areas, but what was gained in quantity was lost in quality.

It is not surprising that children growing up in this environment were poorly fed. They ate a diet composed mainly of bread and dripping, with occasional meat meals. They lived in the squalid narrow streets from which the sun was excluded by the smoke and dust pouring out of the factories. In 1884 a survey of the distribution of rickets in Britain showed that the disease was common in industrial towns, and uncommon in the country. On Clydeside every child examined was found to be affected. Six years later a survey by Dr Thomas Palin showed that the disease was common where sunshine was scarce, and rare where sunshine was abundant. This was a new and unwelcome idea. Eminent physicians who had formed their own, often exclusive, theories were not going to accept such a simple suggestion. The disease must be due to infection, or a disturbance of a gland, or to lack of exercise, they said. With tenacious persistence, each clung to his favourite theory and refused to be shifted, although over the years two theories gained increasing support. These were that rickets was due to deprivation of sunshine, as Dr Palin had suggested, and that it was caused by a defective diet. The latter theory became increasingly popular after Professor Hopkins had written in 1906, 'In diseases such as rickets, and particularly in scurvy, we have had for long years knowledge of a dietetic factor'; and Dr Funk had written in 1914, 'It is very probable that rickets occurs only when certain substances in the diet essential for normal metabolism are lacking or are supplied in insufficient amount. The substances occur in good breast milk, also in cod-liver oil.'

This remark may have stimulated Edward Mellanby in

London to experiment by feeding puppies various diets to see if rickets developed. Puppies were known to be particularly susceptible to rickets. Mellanby approached the problem scientifically. He established a standard diet that regularly produced rickets in puppies, and then added different food substances in turn to see if rickets was prevented. After nearly 400 experiments he was able to report in 1921 that cod-liver oil and, to a lesser extent, peanut oil and butter contained some substance that protected the puppies against rickets. He failed to notice that if the puppies were kept out of doors, rickets was less likely to develop, but he did remark that confinement of the puppies in cages contributed to the development of the disease.

Surprisingly, the suggestion by Dr Funk and Professor Mellanby that cod-liver oil protected against rickets was not new. Folk medicine among people living on the coasts of England, Holland, and France had recommended cod-liver oil as a remedy for rickets for generations! And among the peasants, rickets was never found. In 1921 two American scientists, Drs Shipley and Park, discovered how cod-liver oil prevents rickets. They argued that rickets was caused either by a lack of sunshine, or by a diet that was deficient in an unknown substance, which they called X. This was found in fish-liver oils, and was present in butter, but butterfat contained very little compared with cod-liver oil. Quite soon it was discovered that substance X was a fat-soluble vitamin, which was named vitamin D. Vitamin D, or cholecalciferol, was found in large quantities in cod-liver oil (and in other fish-liver oils).

But why should sunlight also prevent rickets? The answer to that question was also quickly found. Sunlight, by irradiating the skin, causes the body to convert an inert substance in the skin called 7-dehydrocholesterol into vitamin D. In the industrial cities the smoke pall that filled the sky prevented the ultraviolet rays of the sun from penetrating into the streets, and the children rarely, if ever, ate fish-liver oils. The deficiency of calciferol prevented calcium in the diet from being absorbed, mobilized, and deposited in the bones, so that the bones became softer than normal. In infancy and childhood bone growth is rapid, and with a lack of the normal mineralization of bone, the bones softened and became twisted. Rickets developed. This occurred especially when the child began to walk, because the weight of the body on the softened bones led to bowed legs and arms, and to knock-knees. The shape of the pelvis became distorted and, if the child was a girl, this made child-bearing difficult in later life.

Once the cause of the disease had been found, it might be assumed that it would have been eliminated at once. Cod-liver oil is cheap. Yet a survey of infants in 1943 showed that in Leeds, Newcastle, and Manchester, 4 per cent of the children had rickets. In Dublin and Belfast 9 per cent, and in Sheffield 10 per cent, of the infants examined had the disease.

This led to a campaign to eliminate the disease in areas where the hours of sunshine are few and industrial smog considerable. In Britain, with wartime food rationing in operation, pregnant women and young children were given vitamin D capsules, and mothers were advised to put their infants out in the sun when it shone. This has led to the virtual disappearance of rickets in Britain, but recently it has begun to appear again as immigrant children from the sunny tropics adapt to living in the temperate countries of Europe and North America, because they tend to avoid sunlight and often eat a diet relatively low in vitamin D and high in phytate. Rickets also persists in some tropical developing countries where children are wrapped and kept indoors, rather than being allowed to play freely in the abundant sunshine. Some adult women in Asian countries who are kept in purdah develop vitamin D deficiency and softened bones because they are never exposed to sunlight and their diet is deficient in vitamin D. In adult life the disease is called osteomalacia. Osteomalacia may also affect elderly people in the developed countries particularly solitary men living on restricted diets, but it is very uncommon.

In all cases of disease due to vitamin D deficiency, the cure is simple. It is to supply a diet rich in calcium and

··

Good Sources of Vitamin D

Cold water fish (herring, mackerel, salmon, etc.)
Fish-liver oil (especially cod-liver oil)
Liver
Dairy products
Eggs

Most people in Australasia, Europe, and the USA obtain all the
vitamin D they need from the food they eat.

··

phosphorus and to give an appropriate dose of vitamin D
each day.

Today, in most countries young children are exposed to the
sun judiciously; and in countries with a low number of hours
of sunshine, cow's milk fortified with vitamin D is available.
In addition, infants and very young children are usually
given daily vitamin D supplements. Old people would also be
wise to take vitamin D supplements, particularly if they eat a
restricted diet. But perhaps a seat in a sunny corner with a
gossiping friend would be a better way of preventing vitamin
D deficiency.

Most people do not need additional vitamin D, as they
obtain all their requirements from sunshine or from food.

Excessive ingestion of vitamin D, in the false belief that if a
little vitamin does you some good, a lot will do you far more
good, can be dangerous. If too much vitamin D is given to
babies, they lose their appetite, and become irritable and
depressed. An excessive amount of the vitamin causes a
much greater than normal absorption of calcium from the
milk the baby drinks, and paradoxically removes calcium
from parts of its bones, causing a disease. But this is not
usual, and most people affected by excessive vitamin D
intake are adults who have read somewhere that large doses
of the vitamin benefit certain diseases, notably rheumatoid
arthritis. There is no evidence that the vitamin does help, but
people are gullible. The individual who develops vitamin D
toxicity becomes weak and has headaches, tiredness, and

bouts of vomiting and diarrhoea. Later the kidneys may be affected, and if the excessive amount is taken over a long period, the blood vessels may become calcified. Excessive vitamin D can be harmful in another way. It raises the level of the cholesterol in the blood and, as is shown in Chapter 10, high blood cholesterol is a risk factor in coronary heart disease.

The toxicity level of vitamin D varies, but the problem can be avoided by limiting the daily intake to less than 50 µg. The average daily needs of vitamin D for infants and children under the age of 5 is 10 µg, which is also the requirement for pregnant and lactating women. All other people, of both sexes and of all ages, require no more than 2.5 µg a day. Since butter and margarine contain vitamin D, most people obtain all the vitamin D they need from the food they eat, and supplements are unnecessary. In some countries milk is fortified with vitamin D so that vitamin capsules are not strictly necessary, provided children play in the sun.

A Vitamin in Search of a Disease (Vitamin E, or Alpha-tocopherol)

In 1922 a group of research scientists at the University of California fed a colony of rats on a special diet which contained all the nutrients known to be essential at that time. The rats thrived on this diet, but the females failed to reproduce normally, and almost all their foetuses died before birth. When fresh lettuce, yeast, wheat, oats, dried alfalfa, meat, and milk were added to their diet, the females reproduced normal offspring. The inference obviously was that the special diet lacked an essential nutrient, probably a vitamin. Eventually this missing vitamin was identified as a fat-soluble alcohol, and was named tocopherol from the Greek words tocos, meaning childbirth, and phero, meaning to bring forth or deliver.

However, nutritional scientists who used a sequential classification for vitamins, used the term vitamin E to identify the newly discovered vitamin. By 1938 vitamin E, or alpha-tocopherol, had been synthesized in the laboratory and research began in earnest. Diets containing various quantities of vitamin E, or no vitamin E at all, were fed to rats, rabbits, chickens, dogs, sheep, and cattle to see what happened. The results were bizarre and varied quite considerably, depending on the species. For example, when male rats were fed diets deficient in vitamin E, the sperm-producing cells in their testicles degenerated, as did their livers. Chickens developed brain damage, muscular incoordination and eventually paralysis, and calves developed heart disease.

It was argued that if a deficiency of vitamin E caused these serious conditions in animals, a lack of vitamin E might also be the cause of impotence and sterility in men, repeated abortions in women, muscular weakness in both sexes, and might be a cause of coronary heart disease. But over the years, in a wide variety of clinical situations, no adult human given extra vitamin E showed any improvement. It remained a vitamin in search of a disease. This is because vitamin E deficiency is very unlikely to occur, as the quantity needed is readily obtained from many foodstuffs eaten by humans, such as vegetables, fruits, meat, fish, and dairy products.

Vitamin E is not destroyed by cooking, and the normal diet provides for more than the recommended daily requirement of 5–30 mg. Since vitamin E acts as an antioxidant, preventing fats in the body from being broken down by oxygen, the higher intake is needed by people who eat large quantities of fats. It was also discovered that people who ate polyunsaturated fats in preference to saturated fats needed more vitamin E, as polyunsaturated fats are more likely to be oxidized. This led to the suggestion that people who had heart attacks and had been induced to eat margarine rather than butter, and fish in preference to beef, should have vitamin E supplements. The argument was only half true. The fact that polyunsaturated-fat eaters needed a larger daily intake to prevent fat oxidization was true, but since margarine (which is made from polyunsaturated fats) contains nearly fifteen times as much vitamin E as butter, and fish ten times as much as red meat, additional vitamin E supplements are unnecessary.

In order to see if a deficiency of vitamin E harmed man, Dr Howitt, head of the Biochemical Research Laboratories at the Elgin State Hospital in Illinois, was given a commission in 1967 by the US National Research Council to find out what happened to people given a diet containing only one-third the amount of vitamin E found in a typical American diet. The results showed that the low-vitamin E subjects were as healthy and as active in every way as people eating ordinary diets, despite the reduction of their blood plasma alpha-tocopherol by 80 per cent. The only abnormality found was that their red blood cells lived for only 110 days instead of the average of 120 days. Dr Howitt concluded that humans need only a modest amount of vitamin E, and this amount is provided in the diet, even if it is a poor one. He admitted that in exceptional circumstances a deficiency in vitamin E might lead to disease, but it was most unlikely to occur.

In 1967 it did—in exceptional circumstances. In one hospital in the USA premature babies were fed on a synthetic milk substitute because it was believed they would thrive better than if they were given human milk or cow's milk. The mixture contained a higher proportion of protein and a lower proportion of fat. The babies did thrive, but eleven developed a blood disease: haemolytic anaemia, in which the red blood cells live for a shorter time than usual. Investigations revealed that the milk substitute contained very small quantities of vitamin E, and when the babies were given vitamin E supplements, the anaemia was cured. The error was in trying to be clever and giving the babies a milk substitute instead of milk. Babies with the rare congenital disease called cystic fibrosis require extra tocopherol because they are unable to absorb the quantity provided by milk feeds, but for normal babies, human milk and cow's milk contain all the vitamin E they require. However, vitamin E may have a beneficial effect in preventing oxygen-induced damage in premature babies.

For people on normal diets, vitamin E supplements are

unnecessary, despite exaggerated claims, at intervals, that the vitamin improves sexual potency and cures diseases as different as recurrent abortion in women, sterility in men, coeliac disease in children, and diabetes in both sexes. The evidence, after careful study, is that the claims that vitamin E had alleviated any of these diseases are false at best and dangerously untrue at worst.

In recent years a further claim has been made for vitamin E, in what is called a 'thrilling breakthrough in skin care'. It is claimed that vitamin E removes wrinkles, blemishes, dryness, stretch marks, bad odours, and that it rejuvenates ageing skin, as well as heals burns and wounds more quickly. Most of the skin creams and underarm deodorants in which vitamin E is an ingredient are marketed in the USA. With the suspicion that the claims were false, the Consumers' Union of US, Inc. searched all the reputable journals on skin disease and contacted leading dermatologists. In no British or American dermatological journal did they find a single article, report, or letter about vitamin E in the treatment of skin diseases; and not a single dermatologist reported that he or she found vitamin E to be a 'thrilling breakthrough in skin care'. The claims were also investigated by the New York State's Consumer Frauds and Protection Bureau, who enquired especially from the American Medical Association's Committee on Cutaneous Health and Cosmetics. 'To date', reported the chairman in reply, 'there is absolutely no evidence that vitamin E applied to the skin is in any way beneficial to that organ.' As a final check in their investigation, the Consumers' Union telephoned several of the manufacturers. None could refer the investigators to any reported or unreported controlled study of vitamin E's efficiency in skin disorders. The claims were spurious; the advertising, as one marketing director admitted, was 'on the outrageous side'. The same findings were made when the efficacy of vitamin E as an underarm deodorant was investigated: it had no effect.

In the case of skin creams containing vitamin E, all that the credulous consumer loses is cash. In the case of the claims that vitamin E cures heart disease, it could lead heart-disease sufferers to delay obtaining proper medical attention for their condition. This can have serious consequences.

The idea that vitamin E could prevent heart disease was pushed in Canada in 1946 by two Canadian doctors Drs Wilfred and Evan Shute. They were reported in *Time* magazine to have claimed that vitamin E successfully 'benefited four types of heart ailment (95 per cent of the total): arterio-sclerotic, hypertensive, rheumatic, old and new coronary disease. The vitamin helps a failing heart. It eliminates anginal pain. It is non-toxic.' This was good news indeed. Here was hope for millions of sufferers. The Drs Shute's claims were backed by Dr Vogelsang and his colleagues, but all their trials were uncontrolled. When properly controlled scientific studies were made between 1946 and 1973, no trial showed any benefit in the use of vitamin E to treat heart disease.

In a carefully worded statement issued in 1973, the National Research Council of the USA reported that a full investiga-tion of the effects of vitamin E on human health showed them all to be false. Generously, the statement reported that 'many of the claims made for vitamin E are based on misinterpretations of research on experimental animals'. For example, the statement points out that the claim for vitamin E's ability to enhance sexual potency inappropriately stems from research that showed it to be among the factors required to prevent sterility in male rats and to permit normal preg-nancy in female rats. 'Claims that the vitamin prevents heart attacks result from a similar misinterpretation of research' said the statement. 'While a vitamin E deficiency did cause heart-muscle abnormalities in cattle and sheep, similar studies done on monkeys produced no such consequences.'

The statement further reported that the widespread distribution of vitamin E in vegetable oils, cereal grains, and animal fats makes it highly unlikely that humans ever suffer from any deficiency of the vitamin. Additional dietary supplements are therefore considered unnecessary. Vitamin

E is no more a cure for anything than is snake oil or goanna juice. It remains a vitamin in search of a disease.

'Fresh Rice is Never Toxic': The Story of Thiamin

The problem with vitamin B is that it is not just one vitamin but a number of vitamins that have different chemical formulae and different names, and perform different functions in the body. The vitamins that make up the B complex are found in such a variety of foods that it is unusual for people who eat a balanced diet to require vitamin B supplements, although many people take them. It has not always been like this. In the past, deficiency of two of the B vitamins, thiamin (vitamin B_1) and niacin led to severe illness and death.

Until the early part of the nineteenth century most of the people of east Asia ate a staple diet of rice, which was sown, grown, harvested, and milled in the village. Usually the milling was done laboriously in a hand-mill by the women of the family. The work was hard, as the husk was resistant to separation from the grain.

Watt's invention of the steam-engine in England and the technological advances it produced led to the introduction of power-milling. The advantages were considerable. The harvested rice was taken to the mill, the husking was done mechanically, and a fine white, attractive-looking rice was produced; no longer did the women have to spend hours pounding and grinding the paddy. To the entrepreneurs of Asia, and to the European merchants, the new process was financially attractive. Engines made in the West were sold to Asia. European and Asian businessmen set up rice-mills. The better the rice was milled, the more bran there was to be sold for animal food. The more rice that was milled, the more there was available for the urban dwellers, and rural labour could be diverted to other ends such as growing cotton, tea, indigo, and other cash crops, which were sold cheaply to the colonial power, and returned to the colonies as expensive manufactured goods.

The mechanical methods of rice-milling spread through

The B Complex Vitamins

Name	Function	Deficiency leads to	Excess may cause
Thiamin (Vitamin B_1)	To metabolize carbohydrates	Uncommon except among alcoholics	No effect
Riboflavin (Vitamin B_2)	For the body to use proteins; ? to keep the skin healthy	May cause skin lesions	In large injected doses, may damage kidney
Niacin	For the body to use proteins, fats; in large doses, may reduce cholesterol	Pellagra	May disturb heart rhythm
Pyridoxine (Vitamin B_6)	For the body to use protein	? A factor in mood changes	In doses over 100 mg, may cause nerve damage
Cyanocobalamin (Vitamin B_{12})	For the development of red blood cells	Pernicious anaemia	No effect
Folic acid	For the development of red blood cells	Megaloblastic anaemia	No effect

Other B vitamins such as pantothenic acid and biotin are widely distributed in foods, and spontaneous deficiency in humans is not seen. Bioflavinoids, pangamic acid, laetrile, inositol, orotic acid are not vitamins and are not required for good health.

Asia quite rapidly, and so did a new disease, which was called beri-beri because it resembled an older disease of that name.

This disease was strange. It began with increasing fatigue,

a loss of appetite, and heaviness and stiffness of the victim's legs. Labourers found that they tired easily when doing work that had previously been no problem to them, and their legs became stiff and uncomfortable. Later, tingling and numb areas developed on the skin, and the calf muscles became tender. Sleep became disturbed, with long periods of insomnia. Then, gradually, muscular weakness and wasting became apparent. The victim could no longer work, walked with the support of a stick, with a swaying, staggering gait, and eventually became paralysed. In some cases the body became swollen with retained water, and the breathing grew difficult as a result of fluid in the lungs. Finally, the heart failed. This form of beri-beri, which was called wet beri-beri, also affected small infants aged 2 to 4 months, and they died quickly.

The cause of the disease was obscure. Various suggestions had been made, such as an infective source or a toxic substance in the food. In the 1890s the Dutch government sent a team to Java to try to find out more about the disease. At first the scientists thought that beri-beri was caused by an infection. They abandoned this belief after a year or two. Then one of the team, Dr Eijkman noticed a similarity in the symptoms of beri-beri and a disease in fowls affecting their peripheral nerves, called polyneuritis. In 1901 he published a paper connecting polyneuritis with a dietary deficiency, probably something contained in rice husks. He found that if rice husks were added to the food the fowls ate, they did not develop polyneuritis.

Similar research was progressing in the Federated Malay States, where an Institute for Medical Research had been established in Kuala Lumpur in 1900. Research into beri-beri was given priority because it was common and affected many of the labourers living and working on plantations and estates, and those employed to build railways and roads. For example, between 1890 and 1900, 16,000 cases of beri-beri were admitted to the General Hospital in Kuala Lumpur (which served a population of less than 200,000), and one in five died.

In 1907, the Institute began a series of crucial experiments. First they repeated and confirmed Dr Eijkman's research into polyneuritis in fowls. Then in 1907 two scientists began a series of studies which lasted for four years and finally uncovered the cause of beri-beri. The scientists were two young Europeans, Dr Fraser and Dr Stanton.

The first experiment tried to find out, when other factors were excluded or controlled, if people who ate white rice would develop beri-beri and if other people fed on brown rice would avoid the disease. To do this it was necessary to find an isolated spot far away from any village so that infection brought in from outside could be excluded and so that the subjects involved in the experiments would be unable to buy extra food.

At that time the government was building a road in a remote area of the state of Negeri Sembilan and had recruited Javanese labourers for the job. When Dr Fraser heard about this, he obtained permission to try his diets on the labourers. These men were to be the experimental group, and the experiment was to be called the Durian Tipus Project. In April 1907 Fraser and Stanton travelled by train, mule, and foot to Durian Tipus and examined the 300 labourers. None showed any signs of existing or previous beri-beri. The men were provided with a diet of rice, dried salt fish, onions, potatoes, coconut, tea, and salt (which was, in fact, the diet they usually ate) and were divided into two groups. The first group's rice ration was white rice. The second group were given brown rice which is steamed before picking off the husk, some of which adheres to the grain. Each group had to eat the same diet for about six months, and then the groups changed over and ate the other type of rice. The rest of the rations remained identical in both groups.

The first group, eating white rice, remained well until early August. Then the first case of beri-beri appeared. A month later, four more cases had occurred, and by October a further six cases had occurred. The group were then fed brown rice and beri-beri disappeared.

The second group, eating brown rice, remained free from

beri-beri for the entire six months and were changed to white rice in the middle of October. The first case of beri-beri appeared five months later and several more followed in the next month. Dr Fraser wrote, 'The general results lend support to the view that the disease beri-beri as it occurs in the Peninsula has, if not its origin, at least an intimate relation with white rice and justifies further research along these lines.'

For the next three years they continued their research. First they tried to find out if white rice contained a poison, and failing to find one, thought that perhaps white rice was deficient in some protective substance. So they started to work with fowls and after many experiments found that brown rice did have a protective substance which had seeped into the rice from the outer layers of the husk during parboiling. They also found that if the 'polishings' that were left after milling the rice were added to white rice, the fowls remained healthy. It was clear to Fraser and Stanton that, as they reported in 1911, 'These researches, which comprise an unbroken sequence of experiments beginning with rices associated with outbreaks of human beri-beri demonstrated that rice is rendered harmful by the milling and polishing process to which it is subjected in the preparation of white polished rice ... As measures for the prevention of beri-beri in this country, it is recommended that the use of unpolished, or undermilled rice be encouraged among those classes of the community in which the disease occurs.'

The same year, a research chemist called Funk was able to extract a water-soluble substance from rice-polishings that would cure beri-beri. He called it the 'beri-beri vitamin'.

By 1926 the beri-beri vitamin, called vitamin B, had been isolated in a crystalline form, and ten years later it had been made synthetically in the laboratory.

The vitamin, which is now called thiamin, is present in small amounts in all living cells and is consequently found in all natural foods. But because it is not soluble in fat it is absent from butter, animal fats, and vegetable oils. In cereals it is found in the outer layers of the grain, and so whole meal is rich in the vitamin, but white flour is poor. However, in most countries thiamin is added to flour to make up the deficiency.

People in Western nations who eat a normal diet are rarely deficient in thiamin, and beri-beri is unusual. But occasionally cases occur, usually among elderly single alcoholics who live on alcohol and little else.

Research in the past fifty years has shown that there is more than one water-soluble vitamin, but all resemble the original vitamin B in many ways. To date eight vitamins in the B complex have been isolated, although only two are associated with human deficiency diseases. The first of these is thiamin; the second is niacin, which prevents pellagra.

Pellagra is found among maize-eating peoples. Maize, or Indian corn, was unknown in Europe until America was discovered, but there it was the staple cereal. As maize grows quickly and easily in places that are unsuitable for other cereals, it is now grown in Africa, southern Europe, and other countries.

Pellagra first appeared in Spain some time after the Spanish conquistadores brought back the new plant from Peru. For three centuries the cause of the disease was unknown, although in 1735 Dr Gaspar Casal of Oviedo had suggested that the new disease might be connected with eating maize. Around this time a particularly severe outbreak of the disease occurred among maize-eaters in Italy. The disease appeared first in the spring. Exposed portions of the skin, such as the back of the hands, the forearms, and the neck, became red and itchy, and small blisters appeared. The skin then hardened and became tough, blackish, and brittle. After a while the tongue became red and swollen, and diarrhoea developed. In severe cases, the victim's mind became progressively clouded. The disease was called pellagra: the name comes from the Italian words pelle, meaning skin, and agra, meaning sour. Students remember it as the disease with the three Ds: dermatitis, diarrhoea, and dementia.

Since that time thousands of cases of pellagra, some severe

(often causing death), have occurred each spring among maize-eating peasants in southern Europe and the southern states of the USA, as well as in Latin America, India, and southern Africa.

The story of the discovery of the cause of pellagra mirrors that of the discovery of the cause of beri-beri. In the early days most people refused to accept that maize was the cause. In the past, pellagra was believed to be due variously to infection, to poison, to a disease contracted from sheep, to eating raw meat, to bad air, and to misery! The discovery that pellagra was a deficiency disease was the result of the persistent work of an American, Dr Goldberger, in the Deep South of the USA between 1913 and 1938. In a series of experiments he fed dogs on a maize diet and produced a condition called 'black tongue', which he claimed was similar to pellagra. In fact, when he fed the same diet to men, they developed pellagra. He then showed that pellagra could be prevented by the addition of milk and a variety of other foods, particularly liver, kidneys, and fish, and could be cured quickly by giving yeast or yeast extracts. The fact that dogs produced similar symptoms to pellagra gave researchers a suitable laboratory animal on which to test food extracts. By 1937 the cause of pellagra had been found: it was the lack of a water-soluble substance of the B group called nicotinic acid or niacin. Like thiamin, niacin is found in the outer layers of wheat, so people who eat wholemeal bread and a mixed diet are rarely deficient in the vitamin. And in many countries, including Australia, Britain, Canada, and the USA, niacin must be added by law if white flour is used for bread.

The reason maize-eaters develop pellagra is because maize has only very small quantities of niacin, and also is deficient in an amino acid called tryptophan, which the body can convert, to a limited extent, into niacin. Why maize should lack this amino acid is not known, because other cereals such as wheat, rye, rice, and barley contain tryptophan. In areas where maize is the staple cereal, and niacin-rich foods are expensive, vitamin supplements of niacin should be avail-

Good Sources of B Vitamins

Thiamin
(Estimated daily requirement: 0.9 mg)

Whole Wheat, wheat germ
Oatmeal
Fortified breakfast cereals
Marmite (Vegemite, Promite)
Pulses, nuts
Yeast
Brown rice

Riboflavin
(Estimated daily requirement: 1.0 mg)

Foods listed for thiamin
Liver, kidney
Wheat bran
Mushrooms

Niacin
(Estimated daily requirement: 20 mg)

Foods listed for thiamin
Liver, kidney
Bran (wheat, rice)

Pyridoxine
(Estimated daily requirement: 1.5 mg)

Meat,
Fish liver
Whole-grain cereals
Potatoes
Peanuts bananas, avocados

Vitamin B_{12}
(Estimated daily requirement: 1.5 mg)

Liver
Kidney, heart
Meat

Folate (folic acid)
(Estimated daily requirement: 0.2 mg)

Green leafy vegetables
Fruit
Wholemeal bread
Liver, kidney

able, but in affluent societies supplements are not needed.

In the late 1960s large doses of niacin were recommended to reduce high blood cholesterol levels. The benefit of niacin, used alone, for this purpose is doubtful, but used with a cholesterol-lowering drug, niacin may be beneficial. However, if the person is diabetic or a potential diabetic, niacin should not be taken in large doses, as it may make control of blood sugar levels very complicated.

Two other vitamins of the B group are very important, and

their deficiency can cause severe illness. These are vitamin B$_{12}$ and folic acid. These two vitamins are needed for the development of the red blood cells, and deficiency in either or both leads to two types of severe anaemia. Anaemia is discussed in Chapter 12.

The Most Expensive Urine in the World: Vitamin C, or Ascorbic Acid

In 1497 Vasco da Gama sailed from Portugal to seek a passage to the spice islands of the Orient. He sailed south along the unknown coast of Africa, and rounding the southern tip of the continent at the Cape of Good Hope he crossed the Indian Ocean to reach land on the Malabar coast of India. It was the beginning of European expansion into Asia, and the beginning of the colonial exploitation on which the economic growth of Europe was to depend.

Vasco da Gama's voyage was not without suffering. The food on the ships was limited. Dry biscuits, decaying meat, and wine were the staple diet of the sailors. The few fruits that were taken aboard were quickly eaten. By the time the Cape was rounded, half of his crew had succumbed to a strange disease which caused swollen, sore, bleeding gums and patches of spontaneous bruising in their skins. They had developed scurvy. By the time the ship reached India, 160 of the men had died.

Da Gama's successful and innovatory voyage opened east Asia to adventurers and merchants of Europe. The spice islands of the Indonesian archipelago held treasures that enabled Europeans to mask the dull, decayed taste of the meat they ate throughout the long Northern winters. At that time it was necessary to kill the cattle in autumn, as the fodder vanished; but salt meat was dull, insipid, and often rancid. The spices hid the taste. East Asia also had silk and exotic merchandise, which was desired by the rich, and merchants were prepared to risk the capital involved in mounting a speculative voyage because of the high potential profit.

Increasing numbers of ships sailed down the coast of Africa, rounded the Cape, and then sailed north-by-east across the Indian Ocean. And on every voyage a large number of the crew became ill with scurvy, and many died. The crews were expendable, the potential profits were great, and so the voyages and the scurvy continued.

For the next three centuries sailors and others continued to die of scurvy. The disease, according to a ship's chaplain writing in 1740, caused

large discoloured spots, dispersed upon the whole surface of the body, swelled legs, putrid gums, and above all, an extraordinary lassitude of the whole body, especially after any exercise, however inconsiderable; and this lassitude at last degenerates into a proneness to swoon, and even to die, on the least exertion of strength, or even on the least motion. This disease is likewise attended with a strange degeneration of spirits, with shiverings, tremblings, and a disposition to be seized with the most dreadful terrors on the slightest accident.

The cure, when it came, was surprisingly simple. It was to ensure that sailors were provided with fresh vegetables or, failing a supply of these, with the juice of oranges and lemons. That was suggested in the late eighteenth century and was finally confirmed by an experiment in the British Navy. In 1796 the physician of the Channel Fleet was able to write: 'The late occurrences in the Channel Fleet have sufficiently established the fact that scurvy can always be prevented by fresh vegetables and cured effectively by the lemon or the preserved juice of that fruit... Whatever may be the theory of sea scurvy, we contend that recent vegetable matter imparts a something to the body, which fortifies it against the disease.' What the 'something' was remained obscure for over 120 years.

As the disease was apparently confined to seamen on long voyages, and was uncommon in Britain, it did not pose a problem to most doctors. The desire to find what the 'something' was persisted in the minds of a few physicians, but little advance could be made until the accumulation of knowledge in the nineteenth century led to the development of the science of biochemistry. Even then problems remained. Clearly it was impossible to experiment with humans, and no animal apparently developed scurvy when fed a diet that would undoubtedly provoke the disease in humans.

Then in 1907 it was found that guinea-pigs developed the disease when placed on a diet containing no green grasses, vegetables, or fruits. Using various extracts of citrus-fruit juices, which had proved so successful in preventing scurvy in sailors, scientists were able to isolate the protective factor, and it was given the name ascorbic acid because it prevented the scorbutic disease, or scurvy.

Vitamin C, or ascorbic acid, is obtained mainly from fruits and vegetables. Citrus fruits and guavas are particularly rich in the vitamin, as are some green vegetables, such as brussels sprouts and broccoli. The concentration of the vitamin in potatoes is not high, but if large amounts of potatoes are eaten, as in Ireland and Scotland, these tubers can provide most or all of the vitamin C requirements, particularly when boiled in their skins or baked. The amount of vitamin C contained in potatoes diminishes the longer they are stored, so the previous year's crop that is eaten in late spring and early summer before the new potatoes become available may contain very little. Each year occasional cases of scurvy are diagnosed in Scotland and Ireland, usually among elderly men living alone who dislike, or cannot afford to buy, fresh fruits and vegetables.

The quantity of vitamin C available from vegetables and potatoes depends on the method of preparation and cooking. Vitamin C is soluble in water and is destroyed by excessive cooking. Unfortunately, the English way of cooking is to boil vegetables in large quantities of water. Not only does this reduce the original content of vitamin C by about half, but it produces a mushy, soggy end-product.

Apart from fruit and vegetables, other foods contain only small amounts of vitamin C. For example, meat, eggs, and milk contain only minute traces. Luckily, the amount needed to prevent scurvy is small. It is less than 10 mg a day and at least twice that amount is contained in a single orange or other citrus fruit or in 30 ml (1 oz.) of fruit juice. This is exactly the daily ration recommended to the British Navy. An ordinary helping of green vegetables (about 60 g or 2 oz.), if it is not boiled to mush, provides 25 mg of vitamin C, and 120 g (4 oz.) of potatoes provides about the same amount, so a normal diet will protect most people from scurvy.

The body has sufficient stores of vitamin C to last two or three months. To maintain the body stores you need an intake of about 30 mg a day (the amount obtained from a orange). Pregnant women and cigarette-smokers require about 60 mg a day. Some hospital patients who have been operated on need double that amount, as absorption of the vitamin may be reduced, and healing following trauma or surgery requires extra vitamin C.

For nearly all people, the recommended daily amount of 30–60 mg will prevent scurvy and allow for individual variations in the way food is prepared and cooked, and what foods

....

Good Sources of Vitamin C
(Estimated daily requirement: 40 mg)

Vegetables	*Fruits*
Broccoli	Grapefruit
Brussels sprouts	Gooseberries
Cabbage	Kiwifruit
Capsicum	Lemons
Cauliflower	Oranges
Spinach	Papaya (paw paw)
Watercress	Pineapple
	Raspberries
	Rock-melon
	Strawberries
	Tomatoes

An average serving of any will provide all the vitamin C you need for the day. Vegetables should be cooked in the minimum of water or, preferably, steamed until they are slightly crisp, not mushy.

....

are eaten. Most people living in the developed nations eat a diet that provides at least 30 mg, and often more than 60 mg, of vitamin C daily, so that supplements of the vitamin are usually unnecessary, and merely pass through the body to be excreted in the urine.

There are exceptions, however. Elderly people living alone, who have small incomes and limited mobility (and so find it difficult to shop), may become vitamin C deficient and even develop scurvy. Such people perforce tend to buy cheap energy-dense foods and cannot afford fresh fruit and vegetables. As one Australian nutritionist wrote: 'If an elderly person who is on a low intake of Vitamin C develops an infection, the level can drop rapidly to a dangerous low and scurvy may develop.' In addition, those providing them with extra meals may be largely ignorant about nutrition. It is likely that this situation may also exist in countries where dietary habits are similar to those in Australia but where fresh fruit and vegetables are even more expensive and often beyond the reach of the elderly, solitary poor.

To maintain your body's reserve of vitamin C:

- Eat a helping of fruit or vegetables each day.
- Choose food that is in good condition.
- Eat food soon after it is bought, or keep it refrigerated.
- Prepare food near the time you intend to eat it.
- Don't leave vegetables soaking in water.
- If you need to reheat vegetables, use a microwave if possible.

In 1972 Dr Linus Pauling, Nobel prize-winner in Biochemistry, suggested that the recommended daily intake of vitamin C has resulted 'from a concentration by the authorities on the need to prevent scurvy' and that 'we should ask whether larger amounts might not be needed to provide an optimum state of health'. When a scientist of such distinction as Dr Pauling makes that sort of remark, one must review his evidence. In 1969 Drs Chaudhuri and Chatterjee had shown that most animals are able to synthesize vitamin C in their gut.

Only man, other primates, the guinea-pig, the red-vented bulbul, and bats are unable to synthesize the vitamin, and require ascorbic acid in their diet. Linus Pauling argued from this that at some point during the several thousand million years of the evolution of living things, these animals lost their ability to synthesize ascorbic acid because they chose a diet that was rich in the vitamin. Man evolved from the great apes, and the great apes, during the millions of years of their evolution, were and are vegetarian. They eat large quantities of leaves, fruits, grains, and nuts. Dr Pauling has calculated that great apes take in an average of 2,300 mg of ascorbic acid daily, and infers from his evolutionary argument that humans should take in a similar amount each day. If we did this, our state of health, 'including our ability to resist infection such as the common cold', would be greatly improved.

For many years a belief has existed that eating extra fruit will reduce the likelihood of catching colds, and Dr Pauling has made this folk belief scientifically respectable. However, his evolutionary hypothesis is difficult, if not impossible, to test, because of large gaps in the data. But it is possible to assess reasonably objectively whether an increased intake in vitamin C will prevent the common cold, which infects and causes suffering to millions of people each year. Dr Pauling claimed that if a person took 100 mg of ascorbic acid each day the incidence of colds would drop by about 45 per cent. If vitamin C did prevent colds to this extent it would be a medical breakthrough of dramatic proportions, eclipsing almost any other of recent years. In most developed nations huge sums of money have been invested over the past thirty years in research to prevent the common cold, with a monotonous lack of positive result.

At the time Dr Pauling wrote his paper, only four dependable double-blind studies had been reported. In these studies the effect of ascorbic acid in a daily dose of more than 100 mg was compared with a dose of a dummy sugar or citric acid tablet to see which group of people—those taking the vitamin or those taking the dummy—had fewer colds, and if they did get colds, whether these were less severe in one group or the other.

A major problem with this kind of investigation is that the definition of a cold is inexact, and is interpreted differently by different people. A second problem is that the duration of the trial differed in all four investigations and the dose of vitamin C was not identical. Dr Pauling was particularly attracted to the trial made in Switzerland by Dr Ritzel which involved 279 students at a ski-school and lasted a week. Dr Ritzel claimed that the students, who took 1,000 mg of vitamin C each day, had 45 per cent fewer colds than those taking the dummy tablets. The scientists conducting the other three investigations also reported that their results suggested that the people taking vitamin C had fewer colds, but the percentage differences between them and the controls were far less over the longer period of their investigations.

Dr Pauling enthusiastically supported his belief in a book entitled *Vitamin C and the Common Cold*, published in 1970. The book had a wide popular appeal but also received a great deal of criticism from scientists and scientific writers.

Because colds are common and inconvenient and because of the amount of public interest aroused by Dr Pauling's book, groups of scientists in Britain, Canada, Ireland, and the USA have tried to answer two questions: Will large daily doses of vitamin C reduce the frequency and duration of colds? Does vitamin C make you feel better if you do catch a cold?

To provide the answers the trials had to extend for at least ninety days and large numbers of volunteers had to be involved. In addition the trials had to be double-blind. This meant that half the volunteers had to take the dose of vitamin C recommended by Dr Pauling and half had to take an identical-looking capsule, which contained no vitamin C. In the trials the capsules were taken each day, and when the volunteer thought a cold was beginning the number of capsules was increased considerably.

Twenty-three well controlled trials involving over 12,000

volunteers had been reported by 1980, and none have been published since that date. These showed that the answer to the first question, 'Will large daily doses of vitamin C reduce the frequency and duration of colds', was a simple 'no!' In no trial did the volunteers taking vitamin C have fewer or shorter colds than the volunteers who took the capsules that contained only sugar.

The answer to the second question was a very doubtful 'possibly'. In the second of the two Canadian trials conducted by Dr Anderson and his colleagues in Toronto, involving 2,400 volunteers for three months in the winter of 1973, large doses of vitamin C (4–8 g) taken as the cold started appeared to reduce the discomfort, but when they repeated the study a year later, they failed to show that vitamin C had any benefit in reducing the discomfort caused by the cold. Similarly, the trial in the USA involving 311 volunteers, conducted by Dr Karlowski and his colleagues, and that conducted by Dr Michael Carlson in Britain, did not show any difference in severity of or disability due to the cold even when large amounts of vitamin C were taken at the onset of the cold.

It seems from the evidence that vitamin C is useless in preventing a cold and probably of little value in reducing its severity.

In spite of these findings, articles regularly appear purporting to show that vitamin C in large doses will prevent colds (or reduce their duration by a day!). Many people reading this material are persuaded to take large doses of vitamin C, which may be harmful.

Large doses of vitamin C may precipitate demineralization of bones, cause the development of kidney stones, reduce fertility in certain women, or interfere with liver function, so masking the early signs of liver disease. These warnings about high dosages of vitamin C should be heeded.

Despite Dr Pauling's evolutionary approach, careful biochemical investigations have shown that a dose of 1,000 mg daily will produce complete saturation of the tissues, and any dose larger than this is simply excreted in the urine.

In fact, the Canadian researchers who discovered this, Drs Spero and Anderson, wrote: 'In the present state of uncertainty we believe that a regular intake of more than 100–200 mg of vitamin C daily should be discouraged.' 'The only thing conclusively proven is that people who take large doses of the vitamin have a high excretory rate', reported another scientist. 'In fact they probably have the most expensive urine in the world.'

12 VALUABLE MINERALS
••••••••••••••••••••••••••••••

Our body contains a variety of minerals, which have varied
and vital functions. These minerals include calcium, iron,
phosphorus, potassium and sodium. Some occur in tiny
amounts, and are called trace elements. These include
chromium, cobalt, copper, fluorine, iodine, magnesium,
manganese, selenium, and zinc.

**If you eat a varied diet it is unlikely that you will fail to
obtain sufficient of the needed minerals from food, with a
few possible exceptions.**

Apart from copper, zinc, and perhaps magnesium, the
trace elements rarely cause health problems. An excess of
copper and a deficiency of zinc affect a few people. The
accumulation of copper in the liver, in people who have
the rare genetic disease, Wilson's disease, may lead to liver
cirrhosis and liver failure. A lack of zinc in the diet, more
accurately poor absorption of dietary zinc because of a diet
based on wholemeal wheat (which contains a lot of phytate),
causes poor growth and lack of development of the penis
in a few west Asian adolescent males. Most of the body's
small store of magnesium is contained in the bones and
the rest in body cells. Magnesium has been claimed to control or prevent heart palpitations and to improve muscle
performance. Deficiency of magnesium in the body, if it
occurs, is most likely to be among people who are alcoholics.
Magnesium deficiency, it is claimed, reduces muscle strength
and increases the risk of heart attacks. Because of these
claims, some athletes take magnesium supplements, and
some doctors prescribe magnesium for patients who have
cardiovascular problems. The scientific evidence that mag-

nesium helps either of these groups of people (unless they are alcoholics) is scanty, and it is doubtful if magnesium supplements are needed by a person who eats a healthy diet.

Deficiency in the non-trace minerals have much wider health implications. However, with the exception of iron and calcium, most people obtain sufficient of them in their diet.

Deficiency in iron and calcium in the diet over a period of time, particularly in women, may cause health problems of considerable magnitude and lead to morbidity and sometimes to death. Because of this, these deficiencies need to be discussed further.

'For Want of a Nail . . .': Iron

Iron is essential for life. It plays a central role in enabling living cells to obtain the energy they need. In humans, iron forms a complex with a substance called haem and a protein. The product, haemoglobin, is formed in the red blood cells of the body, and acts as the vital carrier of oxygen from the lungs to the tissues and cells. The lungs absorb oxygen from the breathed air into the blood. The oxygen is rapidly taken into the red blood cells, where it combines with the haem to form a stable compound. In this way it is safely transported to the cells of the body to supply their energy needs. Once the oxygen is released from the red blood cells and enters the cells of the tissues, another iron-containing substance— an enzyme—is needed so that the oxygen can release its contained energy. Without iron none of this could happen. Yet the human body contains only about 4 g or ½ oz. of iron—the amount contained in a large nail. Three-quarters of the body's iron is in haemoglobin; a small amount (about 5 per cent of the total iron) is held in body cells, and the balance is stored in special cells found mainly in the liver, the spleen, and in bone marrow. This stored iron is available if new supplies are not available from the food, so that the body has a reserve of the vitally needed iron. The reserve is needed because the human body cannot manufacture iron. We have to obtain the iron we need from the food we eat. The new-born baby starts life with about 300 mg of iron, which it has accumulated from its mother during pregnancy, mostly in the last 10 weeks. From birth onwards, all the iron it needs must come from its food. In the first few months of life, it gets little iron from the milk it drinks, but when the infant starts eating cereals and other foods it begins to absorb more than it loses each day, so that by the time the child has grown to become an adult its body contains about 4 g of iron.

Each day about 1 mg of iron—the amount in a pinch of salt—is lost in the cells that are shed from your skin, your gut, or your hair. But each day iron is absorbed from the diet, and so a balance is maintained.

A woman is at a disadvantage. Like a man she loses iron each day in shed cells, but she loses additional amounts as well. Women menstruate, and menstrual blood contains, on average, about 30 mg of iron, which is equivalent to a daily loss of 1 mg. Moreover, when a woman becomes pregnant she requires more iron. Some of this is given to her foetus, and more is needed because a pregnant woman makes a larger volume of blood in her body and some of this is lost during childbirth. Altogether, pregnancy makes an additional demand of about 500 mg (or about 1/50 oz.) of iron.

In the body, iron is dynamic. The red blood cells, like all other living things, have their own life-cycle. They are made, they live, they age, and they die. A red blood cell has a life of about 120 days so that on any one day 1 in 120 of the 250,000 million of your red blood cells die. Put another way, each day 2,000 million red blood cells die in your body. These dead red blood cells release about 27 mg of iron, which becomes available for the 2,000 million new red blood cells that are formed each day in your bone marrow. Extra iron is needed to compensate for the loss of iron in the shed skin and gut cells, and in women to replace the iron lost in menstrual blood. And, of course, if you lose blood in an accident, or because you have bleeding haemorrhoids or a bleeding duodenal ulcer, you will need additional iron. In the tropics extra iron is needed if you happen to have hookworms. Hookworms fasten on to the gut wall, like leeches fasten on to the skin, and suck blood. It is quite remarkable how much blood is lost as a result of a heavy hookworm infestation. In a study made in Malaya in 1956 it was found that 30 ml (1 oz.) of blood was lost each day if the person had a moderate infestation (500 worms), but it rose to 80 ml (or 3 oz.) a day in heavy infestations of over 1,000 worms.

In Western countries, people who take analgesics such as aspirin regularly to give them a lift or to prevent headaches not only risk damaging their kidneys, but also lose some extra blood, because the analgesic irritates the stomach and slight bleeding occurs.

The iron needed to replace that lost from the body is obtained from food, and the best iron-containing foods are meat, eggs, some vegetables, and cereals. The meat need not be red meat. In fact, chicken contains as much iron as beef, and eggs contain about the same amount (2.5–3.5 mg per 100 g). Cereals such as wheat contain nearly twice as much iron per 100 g as meat, but cereals also contain phytate, which prevents iron being absorbed, so they are less useful suppliers of iron. In fact, in most Western industrialized nations, bread is fortified with additional iron.

Unfortunately, only 5–25 per cent of iron in the food is absorbed; the rest is lost in the faeces. The amount absorbed depends on your sex, the type of diet you eat, and whether you are anaemic. A man eating a typical Western diet (which provides more than 25 per cent of the energy from animal protein) absorbs between 6 and 10 per cent of the iron in the diet, and a woman eating a similar diet will absorb about 14 per cent of the iron. If she is pregnant she will absorb about 20 per cent. People who are anaemic absorb between 20 and 30 per cent of the iron in their food.

In contrast, the vast majority of people in the world eat a diet consisting mainly of cereals, in which animal foods provide 10 per cent or less of the energy. A person eating this kind of diet will absorb far less iron, because most of it is bound to the phytate in the cereal. Five per cent of the iron in wheat is absorbed, about 3 per cent of the iron in maize is absorbed, but only 1 per cent of the iron in rice gets into the body.

It is small wonder that iron deficiency nutritional anaemia is so widespread.

Anaemia

Anaemia, and the use of iron to treat it, has been known for over 2,000 years. The ancient Hindus prepared a mixture called Laula Bhasma by roasting sheets of iron and then pounding them into a fine powder, which was mixed in oil, whey, or milk, and given to cure pallor and weakness. The Greek doctors believed that iron, which was the metal of Ares, the god of war, would give strength to the weak. And the Roman physicians used to allow old swords to rust in tubs of water, bottles of which were then given to patients who complained of weakness or pallor.

But it took nearly 2,000 years before an English physician, Dr Sydenham, recognized that iron cured anaemia, which in those days was called chlorosis, or the 'green disease'. It affected young women in particular. In 1681 Dr Sydenham wrote, 'I comfort the blood and the spirit belonging to it by giving a chalybeate* 30 days running. This is sure to do good. To the worn-out or languid blood it gives a spur or fillip whereby the animal spirits which before lay prostrate and sunken under their own weight are raised and excited. Clear proof of this is found in the effect of steel in chlorosis. The pulse gains strength, the face (no longer pale and deathlike) a fresh ruddy colour.'

Today, among the poor, especially in the hungry developing countries, anaemia is common, although not many young Western women suffer from chlorosis. In some cases anaemia has been aggravated by civilization. When all cooking was done in iron pots, a considerable amount of the iron from the

---

* A chalybeate was a mixture of iron filings steeped in cold wine.

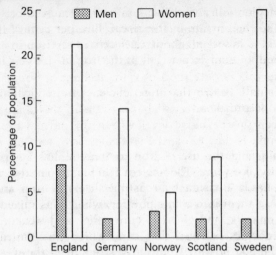

FIG. 12.1. *Anaemia rates in 1980*

pot was eaten with the food. Increasingly, the iron cooking-pot is being replaced by aluminium cooking-pots, and this source of iron has been lost. The value of the iron cooking-pot in preventing anaemia can be judged from the rarity of anaemia among the Blacks in rural South Africa. The Blacks cook their maize in iron cooking-pots, and in addition drink Kaffir beer brewed in rusty iron pots. A South African scientist, Dr Bothwell, measured the iron content in the livers of 147 Black Africans who had died in accidents. In 131 of them the amount exceeded the maximum he expected to find and was far more than the amount found in the livers of Europeans. The Bantu men were certainly not anaemic, and yet from their diet you would have expected them to be anaemic. Dr Bothwell attributed this to the use of iron cooking-pots for food and to the habit of drinking beer which contains a fair amount of iron. Some of the Africans develop signs of iron-overload and become quite ill.

When you want to find out if you are anaemic, the doctor usually takes a sample of blood and measures the amount of haemoglobin in it on a small machine. The result tells him or her the concentration of haemoglobin in a certain amount of blood: a low concentration indicates that the person has anaemia.

Anaemia is only the tip of the iceberg of nutritional iron deficiency. Before the blood shows anaemia, all the stores of iron in the body will have given up their supply to try to keep up the blood level within the normal range. Once anaemia is diagnosed, the stores are low, and the person is truly deficient in iron. To be quite certain of this, the doctor usually does further tests on the blood. The haemoglobin estimation is so easy to perform that a large number of people in a community can be screened to see how common anaemia is.

Investigations made in several European countries in the 1960s have shown that while about 3 per cent of men were anaemic, between 5 and 25 per cent of women chosen from the community at random were anaemic.

The degree of anaemia was usually quite mild, and few, if any, of the women had any symptoms; in fact they all felt perfectly healthy. However, the surveys demonstrate that women, because of menstruation, pregnancy, and lactation, rapidly empty their iron stores and so are vulnerable to anaemia unless they obtain sufficient iron in their diets, or take iron tablets.

In the affluent Western countries it is quite surprising that this can occur. Most Western diets contain between 60 and 90 g of protein, and most protein-rich foods, particularly red meat, are good sources of iron. In addition, complex carbohydrate contains iron. If you eat a good mixed diet, you should obtain enough iron from the food eaten. Women need more iron than men, but even so a woman's average daily iron loss is only 2 mg. This amount is replaced if 11 mg of iron is available in the diet (as only 20 per cent is absorbed from food).

Yet anaemia in women still occurs. This made scientists ask if the diet eaten by many women was providing the necessary amount of iron. In the USA Dr White found that

Good Sources of Iron

(Average daily requirements: males 9–11 mg; females 15 mg)

Food	Quantity	Iron content (mg)
Kidney	100 g	9.2
Liver	100 g	8.8
Oysters	12	7.2
Steak (lean)	150 g	4.5
Fish (fillet)	150 g	2.1
Poultry	150 g	2.1
Egg	60 g	1.0
Breakfast cereal	1 serving	2.5
Bread: wholemeal	1 slice	1.0
white	1 slice	0.4
Potato	medium-sized	0.8
Green vegetables	100 g	1.0
Lentils	100 g	1.8

the average amount of iron in the diet eaten by many girls and women ranged from 8 to 14 mg a day. Surprisingly, he found that among university students the average dietary iron eaten was only 8.5 mg a day. In another investigation of women university students, Dr Monson and his associates found an average daily intake of 9.2 mg of iron. Across the Atlantic, in Göteborg, Sweden, Professor Hallberg reported that an average 15-year-old girl obtained about 11.5 mg of dietary iron a day, and that this decreased to 8.5 mg a day in the diet of elderly women.

It appeared that although iron-rich protein and cereal foods were available, many women in affluent nations were eating diets high in fats and sugar and taking snacks of junk foods rather than eating nutritious foods.

The combined factors of a lack of dietary iron, and the change from iron to stainless steel, aluminium, or glass cooking-pots has severely reduced the iron available among women in two of the richest countries in the world. Over the years this has depleted their iron stores, so that eventually when the women become pregnant or reach their mid-thirties, the symptoms of anaemia appear.

If this is the situation in the rich, industrialized countries of the West, what about the poor countries of the developing world? In these countries only about 10 per cent of the daily calories comes from animal foods, and nearly 80 per cent comes from cereals, usually rice, maize, and wheat, which have a low iron content and contain phytate, which prevents the available iron from being absorbed. The answer to the question is therefore obvious. Large numbers of men and women, and particularly large numbers of pregnant women, are severely anaemic.

This is a serious matter. In an investigation in Malaysia, my colleagues and I found that women who were anaemic in pregnancy were five times as likely to die during pregnancy or childbirth, and were six times as likely to have a stillborn baby or a baby that died in the first weeks of life, compared with non-anaemic women. (There is also some grave concern among paediatricians that babies of mothers who were anaemic during pregnancy may have diminished mental ability because their brains received insufficient oxygen during a crucial period of brain growth). Medical scientists in other countries of the developing world have found a similar, or worse situation.

The World Health Organization believes that anaemia affects over 40 per cent of women in the developing world, if Western standards of diagnosing anaemia are accepted. Among pregnant women the prevalence of anaemia is even higher. Men are less affected and probably no more than 10 per cent of them are anaemic.

This means that more than 500 million people in the world are anaemic. Admittedly, most of them show no signs of anaemia. They are not particularly pale, or weak, or short of breath. They manage to do a day's work. This is because their bodies have adjusted to the lower level of haemoglobin in their blood. But when a stress situation occurs, such as pregnancy, infection, or an accident, they are less well able to withstand it and become much more seriously ill, or may even die. Anaemia is considered by most experts to be partly responsible for the high mortality rates from disease and childbirth found in the developing countries.

This harm to human life could be eliminated easily and cheaply by making iron available. It can be done in two ways. The first way is to make sure, as far as possible, that you and your family eat a diet containing sufficient foods supplying iron to provide about 15 mg a day. As most such foods are relatively expensive, some authorities have suggested that foods, particularly bread, should be fortified with iron. There are problems with this. In contrast to the benefit of adding fluoride to water, which has dramatically reduced the incidence of dental decay (caries), the benefit of fortifying bread with small amounts of iron is doubtful. English medical scientists led by Dr Elwood carried out some very sophisticated investigations into the value of fortified bread. After two years' work, they came to the conclusion that the iron was very poorly absorbed from a normal diet, and if too much iron was added, the flour became rancid quickly. Another investigation in Latin America by Dr Layrisse and his colleagues came to the same unhappy conclusion. Using iron 'tagged' with isotopes and incorporated into various foods, or given as a supplement, they found that an adequate amount of iron would be absorbed from food only if animal protein was eaten as part of the daily diet. Unfortunately, the very people who need the extra iron are those who cannot afford to eat meat except on rare feast days.

A second way to prevent the development of anaemia is to adopt measures that will prevent iron loss from the body as far as possible. Iron loss occurs when you bleed, and in the developed countries there are two main reasons for this bleeding. The first is heavy menstrual periods in some women; the second is, in middle-aged people, bleeding from the stomach or gut. In fact this is the most common reason for anaemia in middle-aged people. Aspirin and other nonsteroidal anti-inflammatory drugs, which are used to reduce the pain of arthritis, may irritate the stomach's lining, leading to a small, undetectable loss of blood (and iron) each day. Haemorrhoids, which are common in middle age, is another reason for blood loss.

In countries outside Europe, North America, Australia, and New Zealand, hookworm is a major contributor to anaemia, as has been mentioned. Another reason for anaemia is bilharzia, caused by a tiny worm which invades the body and enters the blood, after the person has swum or bathed in infested water. From the blood it may infect many organs and tissues. If it damages the bladder, bleeding occurs, with loss of iron. These diseases have specific treatments, and the infected person should also be given iron tablets. As most infected people live in rural areas in the Third World, attempts to eliminate these diseases has hardly touched the surface of the problem, and anaemia continues to be a source of ill health.

Often the lack of one needed mineral or vitamin is found in association with other deficiencies. Iron is no exception. People whose diet provides insufficient iron frequently eat a diet that provides insufficient protein, and certainly insufficient animal protein. The more meat there is in the diet, the better the iron found in other foods is absorbed. People on a poor diet often eat insufficient vitamin C. This applies to the poor of all ages in the hungry developing countries, and in the rich developed countries to the ill, the old, and those on the lowest wages. If the diet does not contain a reasonable amount of vitamin C at the time foods rich in iron are eaten, less iron is absorbed and anaemia may result.

And it doesn't stop there. In the bone marrow, red blood cells are constantly being formed. As they develop they go through a series of changes in shape and size until they are fully mature and are released into the bloodstream to carry out their function of transporting oxygen from the lungs to the tissues of the body. The maturing process takes about ten days and, at a precise time during the growing period, iron is absorbed into the red cells to form the complex oxygen-carrying substance, haemoglobin. As the red cell matures it becomes smaller and a more efficient oxygen-transporter, but it can achieve maturity only if two vitamins are available. These are vitamin B_{12} and folic acid. A lack of the vitamins prevents the cell from becoming fully mature, so that an inefficient, immature cell is let out into the circulation, and because the process is slowed down, fewer cells are let out, and so the person eventually shows signs of anaemia. This anaemia is called megaloblastic anaemia because many of the red blood cells are big (*megalo*) and immature (*blastic*) cells.

Folic-acid deficiency anaemia is the most common megaloblastic anaemia, and it is due to a lack of green leafy vegetables in the diet. The vitamin was first found in spinach leaves in 1941, hence the name folic—from the Latin word for a leaf, folium.

However, the vitamin is found in other leafy vegetables and in liver, kidney, mushrooms, and yeast. In fact it was the discovery that certain women had severe anaemia in pregnancy that led scientists to suspect the presence of the vitamin. In 1931 Dr Lucy Wills was working among poor Hindu women in Calcutta. She noticed that some pregnant women had a severe anaemia, which did not respond to iron treatment. The women were very pale and lethargic and often had swollen legs. Dr Wills reported that they looked as if they had pernicious anaemia but without the nervous signs found in that disease. The anaemia did not respond to the refined liver extract injections that were being used successfully to treat pernicious anaemia, but it did respond to injections of crude liver, or a diet of raw liver. Because the condition resembled beri-beri in some ways, she gave some of her patients yeast extract, which was available as Marmite, and iron tablets. To her delight, the anaemia was cured; in fact the Marmite worked even better than the crude liver injections she had been giving. She wrote a report, which was published in the *British Medical Journal*, in which she speculated that the anaemia was due to a deficiency of an unknown substance, which she believed was a member of the vitamin B group.

It took over twelve years to discover what the vitamin was. In 1943 scientists working in England and the USA isolated the vitamin from crude liver extracts. Oddly, when its chemical structure was worked out it was discovered that it was chemically related to a pigment found in butterfly wings. This gives it its chemical name, pteroylglutamic acid. The human body cannot manufacture folic acid and we have to obtain it from meat, offal, or leafy vegetables, but if these are overcooked, much of the folic acid is destroyed. We normally need only a tiny amount of folic acid each day, and we generally get enough to prevent megaloblastic anaemia. But in pregnancy, women need two or three times as much folic acid, because the vitamin is needed by the growing foetus. And if women do not eat a diet which includes green leafy vegetables, or are not given supplements of folic acid, megaloblastic anaemia may develop with astonishing rapidity. In the affluent nations, folic-acid deficiency anaemia affects fewer than one in every hundred pregnant women, mostly the poorest. But in the hungry developing countries megaloblastic anaemia affects over 5 per cent of pregnant women, and is a hazard to their well-being and to their life.

Vitamin B_{12} is also essential to the proper development of the red blood cells, but it was discovered only in 1948. Nearly a hundred years before that, a physician at Guy's Hospital in London, Thomas Addison, had observed that certain anaemic patients did not respond to iron therapy, but slowly became weaker and weaker, with increasing difficulty in walking, until death eventually occurred after a few years. As Dr Addison could not find a cure for the anaemia, and as it inexorably, perniciously, led to death, he called the disease pernicious anaemia.

For over 120 years, the victims of pernicious anaemia continued to go their slow, painful way to the grave. Then, in 1921 Dr Minot, who was Professor of Medicine at Harvard University, reported that pernicious anaemia could be relieved if the victim ate at least a pound of raw liver each day. It was a desperate cure for a desperate disease. But it did offer hope of survival to the patient, and it gained a Nobel prize for Dr Minot. The biochemists began to work, and soon the huge quantities of liver were replaced by liver injections. But the reason why liver was so effective eluded medical scientists until the 1940s, when two groups, one in Britain and the other in the USA, isolated 20 mg of the active substance from a ton of raw liver. You need only a thousandth part of a milligram of the crystalline vitamin to prevent pernicious anaemia. As the vitamin is found in liver, meat, and dairy products, which most people include in their diet, the disease is uncommon, unless you choose your parents unwisely. People who develop pernicious anaemia have a defect that prevents them from transporting the tiny amount of vitamin B_{12} they need through the wall of their gut. Without the vitamin, the red blood cells cannot mature properly and anaemia results. Furthermore, the vitamin is needed by the nerves, and when it is lacking, various unpleasant nervous disorders result. Today, once pernicious anaemia has been diagnosed it can be treated by injections of a synthetic vitamin B_{12} produced in the laboratory.

Another group of people who may develop pernicious anaemia are strict vegetarians—vegans. Plants do not contain any vitamin B_{12}, and unless the vegan is aware of this he or she may become anaemic quite quickly.

Calcium

Calcium is a vital mineral found in most living tissues. Most of the calcium in the body is in the bones, but its main function is in the tissues and in the millions of cells that make up the body. In the fluid that bathes the cells of the body (and forms 90 per cent of the body mass), calcium (in the form of ionic calcium) maintains the function of the nerves and muscles. Inside the cells of the body, calcium ions help to control the functions of the cells and regulate their response to hormones. Without calcium ions, the messages transmitted by the nerves cannot pass to the cells under their control. Without calcium ions, the cells that secrete hormones and other secretory products are unable to release them.

To fulfil these vital functions, the body keeps the level of calcium in the blood plasma (and in the tissue fluids) in a very narrow range. If the level starts to fall below the range, calcium is released from its stores in the bones. In fact, the bones act as a calcium bank, which contains nearly all the calcium an adult has in the body. The amount of calcium in bone is about 1.2 kg (2½ lb.). When calcium is needed by the body tissues and cells, it is released from the bones by the action of a special hormone. The lost calcium is replaced later by calcium obtained from the food we eat.

Each day, we lose about 1,100 mg of calcium from our body, mostly in the motions (faeces), after passing through the lining of the gut. Calcium is also lost in the urine. Thoughout the day, blood reaches the kidneys in large amounts. In the kidneys, waste substances are filtered from the blood and are passed out of the body in the urine. The calcium in the blood also passes through the kidneys, over 10,000 mg reaching the kidneys each day. Most of this calcium is reabsorbed by the cells of the kidneys and returns to the blood, but about 200 mg is lost in the urine.

Calcium enters the body in the food we eat. Depending on the body's needs, only a portion of it is absorbed through the lining of the gut to enter the blood. This amount of calcium replaces the calcium lost in the faeces and urine, and most healthy people's calcium balance is zero: as much is absorbed as is lost (see Figure 12.2).

An average European diet provides about 1,100 mg of calcium each day, principally in milk and milk products such as cheese, and to a lesser extent in bread (which in Britain has calcium added to the flour to counteract that lost in milling). The diet of most people in the hungry, developing world does not contain much milk, so the amount of calcium provided is lower. In India, for example, an average of 50 mg per head per day is obtained, which is only about one-third of that provided by a European diet.

This is not such a serious situation as might appear.

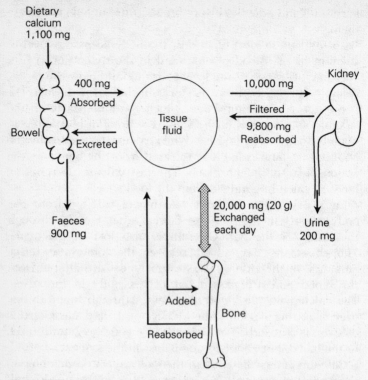

Fig. 12.2. *Calcium metabolism in a healthy diet (mg per day)*

Between 60 and 70 per cent of the 1,100 mg of calcium in the European diet is not available for absorption. This is related in part to the Western diet, which is rich in protein and high in salt, two substances that hold calcium, preventing it from being absorbed. The calcium that is not absorbed is lost in the faeces. A much lower proportion of the calcium in the Indian diet is held and then lost in the faeces so that relatively more is available to be absorbed. In both diets, in general, sufficient calcium is provided by food and is absorbed to replace that lost to the body.

The calcium is absorbed through the cells lining the intestine by becoming bound to protein-carriers, which transport it from the gut into the blood. Before this can happen, there must be a certain amount of vitamin D_3 in the body, as the protein is unable to link to calcium in the absence of this vitamin. When vitamin D_3 is deficient, rickets occurs in children, and the bones of adults become soft and distorted.

The absorbed calcium is transported in the blood and transferred to the bones or, if the blood level becomes too high, is excreted by the kidneys. Although the limits of the amount of calcium in the blood are strictly regulated, a constant exchange occurs from the calcium in the diet into the blood, from the blood to the bones, from the bones to the blood, from the blood to the kidneys, from the kidneys to the urine, and from the urine back into the blood or out into the lavatory pan.

The regulation of this sequence is complex, and scientists are still discovering more about how it operates. Once the calcium has been absorbed into the bloodstream, the regulation of its level in the blood is controlled by two hormones. The first is a hormone produced by tiny glands found in the neck near the thyroid gland. They are called parathyroid glands, and the hormone they produce is called parathyroid hormone. If the blood level of calcium falls, more parathyroid hormone is secreted. This mobilizes calcium from the bones, and by stimulating hydroxy vitamin D (the active metabolite of vitamin D) production in the kidneys reduces the amount lost in the urine. The second hormone involved in regulating the level of calcium in the blood is produced by the thyroid gland and is called calcitonin. Although calcitonin is known to be involved in regulating calcium in bone, how it is involved is so far unknown despite intense research.

These complex interactions could cause problems if anything went wrong, but in healthy people they rarely do, at least up to the time of the menopause. This is because sufficient calcium is obtained from food to keep the blood levels normal without drawing on the calcium stores in the bone. At night a slight problem arises, as most people sleep, not snack, at night. As calcium continues to be lost in the urine, its level in the blood would drop if the parathyroid hormone didn't come into play by removing a small amount of calcium from the bone. But the next day the calcium is replaced from the diet.

Two other groups of hormones are also involved in regulating the loss of calcium from bone. These are the sex hormones. In women the sex hormones, oestrogen and progesterone, are produced by the ovaries. In men the sex hormone androgen is produced by the testicles.

The sex hormones protect the bones from the calcium-extracting effect of parathyroid hormone directly, or indirectly, by increasing the secretion of calcitonin and preventing bone loss.

In most people the system works admirably. The bones, which are constantly being renewed, remain strong and rigid. The diet provides all the calcium needed to keep them strong; there is enough vitamin D_3 to ensure that calcium in the diet is absorbed; parathyroid hormone and calcitonin regulate the level in the body. But certain things can upset this admirable state of affairs. One is reduced mobility; another is the loss or reduction of the sex hormones.

Reduced mobility leads to a loss of calcium from the bone but the effect of the loss of, or reduction in, oestrogen is much more serious. The level of oestrogen in the blood falls dramatically after the menopause. When this happens, first, less calcium is absorbed from the food eaten, and second, the level of calcitonin may fall. The result of these two changes is that to keep up the level of calcium in the blood, the parathyroid hormone takes over to mobilize calcium from the bones, with the result that over a period of time bone tissue is resorbed. This leads to a reduction in the bone mass.

Bone

During our growing years, calcium is steadily absorbed from the food we eat to maintain a constant level in the blood and to supply the needs of the growing bones. Once we stop growing, the amount of calcium in the bones levels off, and remains at 1.2 kg until the age of 40 in women and about thirty years later in men.

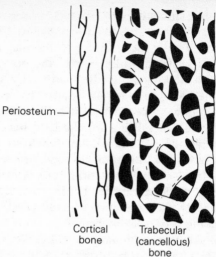

Periosteum —

Cortical
bone

Trabecular
(cancellous)
bone

FIG. 12.3. *The structure of a long bone*

Everyone knows what bones look like—they are hard, shiny, shaped objects, which do not decay like the rest of the body after death, but persist for years. From this, one might infer that bone is a static, stable tissue and remains unchanged once a person is fully grown.

Nothing could be further from the truth. Bone is almost as dynamic as skin. It is constantly dying and being replaced. Bone is resilient and is constantly adjusting its structure to meet new stresses. In other words, it is remodelling. Bone has a remarkable plasticity. It has these properties because of its structure and its chemical composition. Its structure comprises a covering of membrane, called periosteum, under which lie numerous blood vessels. Directly beneath the periosteum, there is a dense outer layer of compact bone (the cortical layer), which varies in thickness in different bones. The stronger the bone has to be, the thicker is the compact layer. For this reason, the bones of the arms and legs have thick compact layers, because of the stresses they undergo, when the muscles attached to them contract. The compact bone encloses a small meshwork of spongy bone, which is made up of fine spikes of bone carefully arranged in ties and struts to give the bone stability when it is stressed by crushing or tearing. This is the spongy or trabecular layer of bone (see Figure 12.3). Inside this layer of the bones of the legs and arms is a hollow space filled with bone marrow. The vertebrae, the neck of the femur, and the wrists do not have the central hollow space. Instead it is filled with trabecular bone. The vertebrae differ from the long bones in another way. Although the spinal column, which is made up of vertebrae, carries the weight of the body and needs strength, the cortical layer of each vertebral bone is rather thin, the vertebra being made up mostly of spongy bone. However, the cubical shape of each vertebra gives strength to the spine without making it impossibly heavy.

The basic substance of bone is collagen. Both the compact and the spongy layers of bone are made up of special bone cells, which secrete the protein, collagen. Collagen is an insoluble protein, which forms long fibrous, rope-like, tough strands. These fibrous strands are embedded in a mesh of other organic components, which add to the strength of the collagen.

Collagen is relatively plastic. To give bones rigidity and strength, it is impregnated (saturated) with lime salts, mainly calcium. If a piece of bone is placed in a weak acid solution, the calcium dissolves but the bone retains its shape, as this is dictated by the collagen framework. But now it can be twisted into knots or cut with a knife.

When a fragment of bone is examined under a microscope, its structure is shown. Compact bone consists of layers of collagen impregnated with calcium, rather like the coats of an onion. Bone cells called osteoblasts produce collagen (which is also called osteoid). These cells lie in the bone between the periosteum and the compact bone. Other bone cells called osteocytes are also present and are found between the layers of bone, looking like plum stones. They are derived from some of the osteoblasts and may contribute to the strength of the bone. Osteoblasts (in association with cells called osteoclasts) cause calcium to be deposited

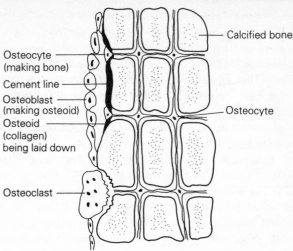

Calcified bone

Osteocyte
(making bone)

Cement line

Osteoblast
(making osteoid)

Osteoid
(collagen)
being laid down

Osteocyte

Osteoclast

FIG. 12.4. *How bone is remodelled*

through the collagen to produce a cement. In the spongy layer the collagen has a different distribution, being laid down in a complicated manner, which may be described as a complex honeycomb. The walls of the honeycomb are formed from collagen and impregnated with calcium, which gives the bone rigidity.

When bone dies or is changed in shape because of microscopic damage, or the need to adjust to new stresses on it, it is said to be remodelled. The remodelling of bone goes on all the time. Each year about 10 per cent of cortical bone and 40 per cent of trabecular bone is remodelled. Bone is first removed by the osteoclasts to a variable depth, depending on the particular bone being remodelled. The removal process (which takes about two weeks) ends when a line of tissue, consisting of collagen, and called the cement line, is laid down. On this cement line the osteoblasts lay down osteoid, which is then impregnated with calcium so that new bone is formed (Figure 12.4). This process, which occurs in all parts of the bones, takes about twelve weeks in young people. As a person grows into late middle and old age, the process takes longer, less new osteoid being formed each day, and so the process may take from sixteen to twenty-four weeks to complete. During this time, in older people, the new osteoid formed is insufficient to replace completely the old bone that has been removed. At first, the young osteoclasts are beneficial, co-operating with osteoblasts to lay down calcium in the osteoid, which converts it into bone. Later the osteoclasts absorb bone, as just described.

This balanced process may become unbalanced in two ways. In the first way, the osteoblasts fail to make sufficient osteoid. The second way in which imbalance occurs is when the osteoblasts have a shortened life-span, and die or are converted into osteoclasts before they have laid down much bone. If these changes occur, less bone is made than is removed and osteoporosis develops. These changes occur as a person grows older.

Bone changes with ageing

Until the age of about 30 in women and later in men, more bone is made than is lost each year, provided you are healthy, eat a diet rich in calcium, and have chosen the right parents! This bone constitutes the bone bank. The maximum size of the bone bank depends on your genetic inheritance, and on the quantity of calcium you have eaten each day from about the age of 15. The bank will be bigger if your diet contained a sufficient amount of calcium—about 1 g a day—in the years between 15 and 30. At age 30 or thereabouts your bone bank has reached its maximum size. For the next few years, probably until you are 40, the bone bank remains at the same size, but then, in women particularly, it begins to decrease, as each year more bone is lost than is made.

At first, in both sexes the loss is small, probably less than 0.5 per cent per year, but when the woman reaches her menopause, the rate of bone loss may increase up to 8 per cent or more each year. Not all women lose bone after the menopause at the same rate. One woman in four loses no more than she did in the years after she reached the age of 40

(0.5 per cent per year). But the remaining three-quarters of menopausal women lose bone at a higher rate. About a quarter of the women lose bone at the rate of 1 to 2 per cent, but the rest lose much larger amounts each year. This increased loss continues for ten years after the menopause when, for some reason, the rate of loss settles down to the rate of loss in the years before the menopause—about 0.5 per cent each year.

The bones of the woman who loses bone at the higher rate will become less dense and more brittle. An unexpected fall or a sudden stress on the brittle bone may lead to a fracture, and the diagnosis of osteoporosis.

Most of the fractures occur in the vertebrae, which make up the spine. At first, inside the vertebra some of the complex network of struts which makes up the trabecular bone break, and the bone slowly becomes more brittle. Later, when sufficient struts have broken, the bone suddenly collapses, and the woman may complain of back pain. If several vertebrae collapse the woman will become stooped and develop a 'Dowager's hump' (Figure 12.5).

Loss of bone also occurs in the bones of the arms and legs. These bones have a thick outer layer, called the cortex, which becomes thinner and more brittle as a person ages. If a post-menopausal woman trips and puts out a hand to save herself, she may fracture her wrist. Later in life, particularly after she reaches the age of 70, when falls are more likely, she may trip and fracture her thigh bone—a so-called fractured hip.

The reason why different women lose bone at different rates after the menopause is unknown, but investigations have shown that women whose mothers had osteoporosis, who are thin, who smoke, and who have to take certain drugs (such as corticosteroids for an illness) are more likely to develop clinical signs of osteoporosis.

Men are not affected so early or so severely. This is because men have a larger bone mass (a bigger bone bank from which to draw without making the bone less dense) and do not experience the hormonal changes that accompany a woman's menopause. In consequence, they do not have

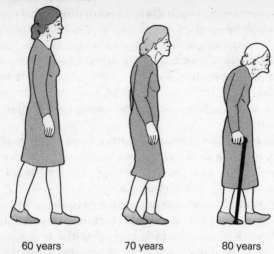

60 years   70 years   80 years

Fig. 12.5. *The 'burden of the years'*

an increased rate of bone loss until they reach the age of about 70.

After this age men and women lose bone at about the same rate, and both sexes may have a hip or a wrist fracture, but women are more likely to have one or other than men.

Osteoporosis is not only incapacitating and painful; it is also very expensive to the community. In 1990 over 1 million fractures due to osteoporosis occurred in the USA. Over half were fractures of the vertebrae, and 200,000 were hip fractures. In Britain 50,000 hip fractures occurred in 1990, and in Australia 10,000 people fractured their hip.

Many of these fractures could have been prevented if action had been taken to build up the bone bank, so that there was more bone to draw on as the person grew older and was losing more bone.

Preventing osteoporosis

As calcium is so important in making the bones strong, and as the bone bank is added to up to the age of 30, the time to

start preventing osteoporosis is in adolescence and the young adult years. From the age of 12 to 30, both men and women would be wise to ensure that they have a daily intake of 800 to 1,000 mg of calcium. It is not difficult to obtain this amount of calcium in the diet.

The richest sources of calcium are dairy products, and smaller amounts occur in green vegetables, and some fruits. A problem arises which affects young women more than men. Many young women choose not to eat dairy products because they do not want to get fat. They can still obtain sufficient calcium from their food if they avoid full-cream milk, and drink low-fat milk or eat yoghurt instead.

Once the bone bank has reached its maximum (at age 30), and loss is beginning, it is uncertain whether a large daily intake of calcium has much benefit in preventing bone loss, or restoring bone, but it will do no harm for you to continue eating a diet containing 800 to 1,000 mg of calcium.

The reason why increased bone loss occurs after a woman's menopause is because her ovaries no longer produce the female sex hormone, oestrogen, which protects against bone loss. But a menopausal woman can prevent the inevitable

....

Good Sources of Calcium

Food		*Amount of calcium (mg)*
Milk (including skimmed)	(250 ml)	290
	(200 ml, 1 glass)	230
Milk (low-fat)	(250 ml)	400
Yoghurt	(200 g)	380
Cheese	(30 g)	260
Cottage cheese	(100 g)	75
Canned salmon	(100 g)	180
Broccoli	(1 serving)	100
Most other vegetables	(1 serving)	40

....

bone loss if she choses to take oestrogen to replace that which is no longer being produced in her ovaries. This is hormone replacement treatment and it is the most effective way of preventing osteoporosis. Nevertheless, it is important that both women and men should also modify other life-style habits. For example, you should:

- take regular weight-bearing exercise, such as walking, three times a week;
- stop smoking, if you are a smoker;
- drink no more than six cups of tea or coffee a day;
- limit the amount of alcohol you drink (see Chapter 9).

These measures will do much to reduce the chance that you will develop osteoporosis, with all its physical and financial consequences.

13 EATING FOR HEALTH

• •

> The twin objectives in devising a diet for the treatment
> of obesity are that it should be effective in removing
> excess fat and that it should become a permanent eating
> habit.
>
> John Yudkin, 1974

The information presented in this book should make it clear
that the diet of most of the people who live in the developed
world is a factor in a number of common diseases. If you
modify your choice of food to eat what Americans call a
more prudent diet, you will reduce your risk of developing
coronary heart disease and stroke, bowel cancer, certain
bowel disorders (notably constipation and haemorrhoids),
and osteoporosis (particularly if you are a woman) and
diabetes in middle age, and, if you limit your alcohol intake,
you will reduce the risk of developing an alcohol-related
disease.

You can change your diet without distorting your food
habits and choices too much. By changing to a prudent diet
you can enjoy a wide variety of foods that are palatable and
probably healthier.

There are two main groups of people to consider: those
whose weight is within the desirable range (that is their body
mass index is 19 to 24.9) and those who are overweight or
obese. This second group can be subdivided into the overweight (BMI 25 to 29.9, over 90 per cent of the group), the
moderately obese (BMI 30 to 39.9, 9 per cent of the group),
and the severely obese (BMI 40 and over, 1 per cent of the
group).

If your weight is in the desirable range (BMI 19–24.9) a

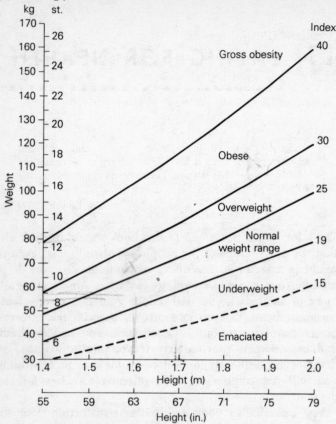

FIG. 13.1. *The body mass index*

sensible, prudent diet, which does not disturb your enjoyment of food to any great degree, will help reduce the risks to your health that have been discussed in earlier chapters.

If you are overweight (BMI 25–29.9) you may want to eat a weight-reducing diet to bring your weight into the desirable range and to maintain it in that range. This has the benefit of reducing the increased risk of developing several illnesses, but whether or not you choose to lose weight depends on you. Unless you are motivated to lose weight, it would be better for you to maintain your present weight.

A Prudent Diet for Health

The following guide-lines should enable you to devise a diet that is healthy and well balanced nutritionally. The principles of the prudent diet have been stated by expert committees in most of the countries of Europe, North America, Australia, and New Zealand.

It is recommended that you should:

- Choose a nutritious diet from a *variety* of foods (see Figure 13.2).
- Eat more foods that contain complex carbohydrates (such as bread, cereals, vegetables, and fruits). Wholemeal bread is preferable to white bread because it contains more dietary fibre, but if you do not like wholemeal bread, eat white bread. Complex-carbohydrate foods should provide over half of your energy needs.
- Try to eat about 120 g (4 oz.) or more of green leafy vegetables and some fresh fruit most days.
- Avoid eating too much fat. Preferably, reduce the amount of saturated, largely animal, fat that you eat (including hidden fat in cakes, pastries, biscuits, and most ice-creams), so that saturated fat supplies no more than 10 per cent of your energy needs. But your total fat intake should make up between 25 and 35 per cent of your energy needs. You can achieve this by:

  eating fewer (and on most days no) pastries, cakes, and biscuits, and not too much ice-cream;
  choosing *lean* meat (beef, lamb, pork) or poultry (removing the skin alter cooking), and eating fish (at least once a week if you can afford it). You should grill, boil, or steam the meat and fish. You should not fry the meat or fish, and should avoid batter;
  reducing the amount of butter you eat or choosing a polyunsaturated margarine. This will reduce the amount of cholesterol that you eat.

- Avoid eating much refined and processed sugars (you could, for example, stop adding sugar to tea and coffee), and choosing sweet drinks.
- Eat some cheese or drink milk (which can be low-fat) either in tea, coffee, or in foods, to give you a reasonable intake of calcium.
- Use less salt. An easy way of doing this is to avoid adding salt to your food on the plate.

- Limit your alcohol consumption.
- Reduce the supply of energy (kilojoules, kilocalories) in the diet in some cases so that your weight remains in the desirable range and your body mass index is 19 to 24.9.

Within these guide-lines it should be possible to buy an interesting variety of foods and devise dishes that are palatable and varied.

If you eat these foods and are in good health, you do not need vitamin or mineral supplements: save your money!

....

If you are moderately (BMI 30–39.9) or severely obese (BMI 40 and over), there is a stronger reason for trying to lose weight, as the risk to your health is greater.

Most people who are overweight or moderately obese want to lose weight not for medical but for cosmetic reasons. They believe that if they lose weight they will be happier about their body shape and image, less depressed about life, and perhaps healthier.

Those whose weight is in the desirable range (BMI 19–24.9) will be healthier if they choose to eat the prudent diet outlined above. Many overweight people (BMI 25–29.9) may also choose to eat the diet, while others will want to reduce their intake of fats and sugar to lose some weight. The prudent diet is easy to follow and is nutritious.

Losing Weight

Four principles of weight reduction:

- Unless the weight-reducing diet is nutritionally sound, easily understood, acceptable, and substantially reduces the amount of energy provided by food, it will fail.
- The diet must permit you to join your family at meal-times and to eat many of the same foods.
- You will need continual support and encouragement to resist the urge to eat.

- You must accept that weight reduction is a slow process, and guard against becoming despondent when the weight loss appears to have ceased.

If you are obese, that is your body mass index is 30 or more, losing weight and keeping to your new lower weight is not easy to achieve, but you will go a long way to achieving it if you follow these principles. Obviously, the greater your initial weight the harder it is and the longer it will take to lose weight. Before you start on a weight-reduction programme, it would be wise to consult a physician to make sure that a reduction in weight is medically desirable and psychologically wise. This raises the question whether obesity should be treated at all. From a health viewpoint, if you are overweight (BMI 25–29.9) and have no evidence of heart disease, high blood pressure, or diabetes, there is only a small health benefit in losing weight. There is a stronger reason if your weight is in the lower zone of moderate obesity (BMI 30–35), and a fairly compelling reason if it is above that (especially if the BMI is over 40), because of the increased hazard to your health.

From the social viewpoint, however, if you are overweight or obese, losing weight may give you a better feeling about your body image.

There is a dilemma in the treatment of obesity: many people start trying to lose weight, but few succeed. After a year of trying to lose weight, only 5 per cent of those dieting will have lost more than 20 kg, and only 10 per cent more than 10 kg. The others may accept that they have failed, or the failure may cause depression.

Unless you are severely obese, the decision to lose weight should be based more on a desire to look 'better' and to feel that it would improve your body shape, than on the increased health risks of obesity, because the risks are perceived as being in the future and are only risk *factors*: they do not mean that you *will* develop the disease. They only say that you are at greater risk than a non-obese person of developing the disease. In other words, the choice to lose weight must be yours, not a decision imposed on you by family or health professionals.

If you are trying to lose weight, you should bear in mind that after the first few weeks of the chosen programme, when you may have lost 2 to 4 kg (4–8 lb.), the average weight loss is between 0.5 and 1.0 (1 to 2 lb.) a week. Most sensible weight-reducing programmes are designed to help you achieve this small but steady loss of weight. Another thing to bear in mind is that a diet sheet alone is not enough. It is less important than your motivation, persistence, and endurance to resist the urge to eat, and to take exercise.

You may recall that the excess energy that you have accumulated over the years is stored in your body in the adipose tissue and in the glycogen–water pool. If you starve, or reduce your energy intake to a very low level (as in a crash diet), you will first extract energy for bodily functions from the glycogen–water pool. The size of the pool varies, but three-quarters of it is composed of water. In non-obese people it weighs about 3.5 kg (7¾ lb.), of which about 1.25 kg is glycogen. In obese people it weighs about 5.5 kg (12 lb.), of which about 2 kg is glycogen.

The glycogen–water pool contains about 17,000 kJ (4,000 kcal) of energy per kilogram of glycogen. When the energy is released from the glycogen, water is also lost. For every kilogram of glycogen used to provide the needed energy, 3 kg of water is lost to the body in urine, sweat, and in the breath. This means that in the first weeks of a very severe reducing-diet (providing less than 2,500 kJ (600 kcal) a day, or in starvation, a fairly rapid loss in weight will occur as the energy available from the glycogen–water pool is used up and a large quantity of water is lost to the body. Within four weeks the glycogen–water pool will be depleted, and a weight loss of 3 to 6 kg (6½ to 13 lb.) will have occurred. By now you will be rather dehydrated and will retain more of the water you drink, and so your weight may increase a bit.

After this time on a starvation diet, any further loss in weight will come from burning up the adipose tissue to release energy from the stored fat. This produces a slow, steady loss of weight. The amount lost weekly will depend on the severity of the restriction of the energy intake, but usually does not exceed 0.5 to 1 kg (1–2 lb.) a week.

If you choose to reduce your food intake sensibly rather than starving or adopting a very-low-energy diet, and choose not to eat high-density foods, that is fatty and sugary foods, you will lose less of the glycogen–water pool, as fat in the adipose tissue will start being used up earlier. The initial weight loss will be less, but much better from a metabolic viewpoint, as the weight loss will continue steadily, even if slowly.

Weight loss is a slow process. For example, take the case of a woman in her forties who is severely obese (BMI 42) and wants to lose 35 kg (77 lb.). The energy equivalent of 35 kg of fat is 1,300,000 kJ (315,000 kcal), as each kilogram of fat contains 29,300 kJ (7,000 kcal) of energy. If she eats a balanced diet that provides 4,620 kJ (1,100 kcal) of energy, and keeps to it, she will have an energy deficit of about 5,000 kJ (1,200 kcal) a day. It will take her a year to lose the 35 kg, but the rate of weight loss will depend on her resting metabolic rate and her lean body mass. The more lean body mass you have (simplistically, the muscle mass and the bone mass), the less adipose tissue you have, and the less fat you have to lose. The higher the metabolic rate, the quicker will weight loss occur, and so the time taken varies. Thus only a range of time can be given to an individual, unless research laboratory facilities are available to calculate the resting metabolic rate and lean body mass.

Weight loss is not easy, and those who decide to try and lose weight can be helped by two strategies. The first is to eat less and to resist the urge to eat. A second strategy is to take regular, fairly strenuous exercise in addition to dieting. You should decide on your strategy first before choosing a weight-reducing programme.

Energy intake (kJ)	Energy expenditure (minutes)			
	Walking	Bicycling	Swimming	Jogging
400	20	14	14	10
600	30	20	20	15
800	40	28	28	20
1,000	60	35	35	30

Exercise as a Means of Losing Weight

Lack of exercise—sloth—is recognized as a factor that may make obesity worse or hinder weight loss. The more exercise you take each day, the less energy is left from your daily intake to convert into fat. Unfortunately, you have to be very active to use up the excess energy (excess, that is, to the body's basic needs) obtained from food. For example, a serving of breakfast cereal with milk provides about 700 kJ, an orange 150 kJ, and a slice of bread and butter or margarine about 800 kJ.

However, regular exercise, especially if taken after meals, may help you lose weight more rapidly and maintain a lower weight, although this seems to vary from person to person.

In addition to a prudent diet, physical exercise improves physical fitness and helps weight loss. You should choose an exercise that you enjoy, and do it regularly.

A Weight-Reducing Programme

What is a weight-reducing programme and how is it different from a slimming diet? A slimming diet usually demands that you alter your eating behaviour considerably, which makes it difficult to keep to the diet for long, with the result that you put on weight again.

Most slimming diets fail after the first few weeks. This has been discussed in Chapter 3 but two points need to be mentioned again.

- Crash diets do not work. Initially, these diets, which provide less than 2,100 kJ (500 kcal) of energy a day, produce a rapid weight loss, but before long you will find it very difficult to keep to the strict, dull diet, and when you stop you usually overeat. Furthermore, if you persist with the diet, semi-starving yourself for a month or more, your body reacts by reducing the metabolic rate by up to 40 per cent. This means that less energy is burned up than if you were eating a diet that provides about 5,000 kJ (1,200 kcal) a day, and the weight loss is rapidly reduced. This is very discouraging, and you will probably abandon the diet.

....

Problems of Dieting

- Dieting is stressful, as the amount of food you eat has to be kept under strict control, and you have to make decisions all the time about how much, what, and how often you should eat.
- You have to stop responding to hunger cues, which may add to the stress.
- Because dieting is stressful, the stress may encourage you to eat more than your diet allows, to compensate for the stress.
- When you eat you may have an intense desire to eat more, and your resolve to keep to your diet may be undermined.
- When you think that you have 'blown' your diet (even if you haven't), you may decide to go on eating because once you start you can't stop. You may tell yourself that although you have eaten too much today, you will keep to the diet tomorrow, but tomorrow never really comes.
- Many dieters have concepts about 'good' food and 'bad' food that may not relate to the food's energy content.
- Because weight loss is slow over the long term, you may be tempted to give up.
- Dieters put on rigid diets find it difficult to eat with friends, or at a social occasion, because it is hard to refuse offers of food, particularly when everyone else is enjoying it.
- If you are on a very strict diet, such as a very-low-calorie diet, you tend to fantasize about food and eating. This makes it even more difficult to keep to the diet.

....

- Crazy diets, which alter your eating behaviour drastically, do not help you lose weight and remain at the lower weight permanently. They may seem to work for a short period, but sooner rather than later you will find that you cannot keep to the diet.

The idea of the weight-reducing programme is that you modify your diet by eating less food, particularly fats and simple carbohydrates (sugar and sugar-containing foods), rather than stick to a rigidly prescribed diet. What you need if you want to lose weight, and to maintain a lower weight, is to reduce your energy intake permanently. The weight-reducing programme aims to do this by changing, but not distorting, your eating habits. It does not rely on simply giving you information as to what you should eat to lose weight, but includes advice about how you can keep to the decision to eat less and still maintain good nutrition. The principles of a weight-reduction regimen are:

- eat less, aiming for 4,200–5,000 kJ (1,000–1,200 kcal) a day;
- aim for a weight loss of about 2 kg a week for the first two or three weeks, then 0.5–1.0 kg a week;
- eat three meals a day, choosing from a variety of foods in the four main food groups: cereals and bread; vegetables and fruit; meat, poultry, and fish; dairy products;
- remember that your eating habits need to be changed as much as your food intake needs to be reduced;
- increase the amount of exercise you take each day (exercise increases weight loss, and may cause metabolic changes that enhance further weight loss).

The programme is based on a nutritionally balanced diet, comprising complex carbohydrates (64 per cent), protein (29 per cent), and fats (7 per cent), which provides about 5,000 kJ (1,200 kcal) of energy intake a day. This is the ratio of foods (with rather more fat) that expert committees recommend for a person whose weight is in the desirable range (see Figure 13.2). The foods provide sufficient dietary fibre, vitamins, and minerals, and so supplements are not usually needed.

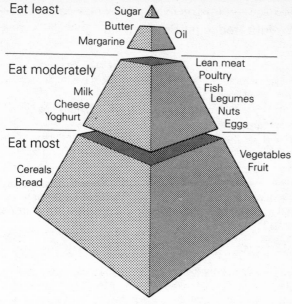

Eat least · Sugar · Butter · Margarine · Oil

Eat moderately · Milk · Cheese · Yoghurt · Lean meat · Poultry · Fish · Legumes · Nuts · Eggs

Eat most · Cereals · Bread · Vegetables · Fruit

FIG. 13.2. *The healthy diet*

The weight-reducing programme is based on three principles:

1 It is effective in burning off excess fat, and provides a good amount of complex carbohydrate (175 g), protein (78 g), and dietary fibre (35 g), and only a small quantity of fat (20 g).
2 The foods that you choose are palatable, and so you can enjoy what you eat.
3 The programme avoids distorting your eating habits as far as possible, for example, you continue to eat three meals a day. This leads to a more rapid weight loss than if you eat only one meal a day (as some diets recommend), because smaller meals eaten more often induce a greater production of body heat (by burning stored energy), which is then dissipated into the surrounding air.

··

The Weight-Reducing Programme

Daily allowances

Bread, preferably wholemeal: 4 × 35 g (1¼ oz.) slices

Rice, pasta, or potato: 60 g rice (boiled), 60 g pasta (boiled), or 1 large (2 small) potato (boiled or baked)

Milk: skimmed (600 ml, 1 pint) or low-fat (400 ml, ⅔ pint)

Butter or margarine: 15 g (½ oz.)

Water, mineral water, tea, coffee: unlimited quantities

Meals

Breakfast

1 orange, ½ grapefruit, or 100 ml (3½ oz.) of fresh orange juice

Bread from the daily allowance or ½ cup cereal (equal to 2 slices of bread)

Main Meals

Meat 60 g lean beef (minced or steak), lamb or pork liver, kidney, tripe, or tongue

or 60 g chicken, duck, or turkey (with skin removed), rabbit, hare, or pheasant

or 60 g fatty (oily) fish, e.g. herring, kipper, mackerel, salmon, trout, sardines, or pilchards (with oil or tomato sauce discarded), or of shellfish

or 90 g of white fish, e.g. cod, flounder, halibut, John Dory, lemon sole, ling, plaice, turbot, whiting. MEATS AND FISH MAY ONLY BE GRILLED OR STEAMED; NOT FRIED

or 50 g cheese (no more than 4 times a week)

or 2 eggs (no more than 3 times a week)

Vegetables As much as you like at each of the two main meals of asparagus, artichokes, cabbage, cauliflower, lettuce, cucumber, beans (French, runner, or baked), broccoli, brussels sprouts, leeks, spring greens, mushrooms, spinach, tomatoes

or 50 g (1½ oz.) beans (butter, haricot, red kidney), carrots, peas, sweet potato, swedes, turnips

Fruit 1 orange, tangerine, mandarin, or 1 apple; or ½ grapefruit, mango, peach, pear, or plum

or 100 g (3½ oz.) of any soft fruit, melon, and ⅓ of an average-sized papaya

or 50 g grapes or ½ a banana

Prohibited foods
  Alcohol (a glass of wine or a light beer adds 340 kJ (80 kcal) to your
     energy intake)
  Sugar, sweets, chocolate, jam, honey
  Canned fruit
  Pastries and puddings
  Milk shakes; cordials; and soft drinks, except for soda water and
     sugar-free soft drinks
  Sauces

....

However, some changes in eating habits and in physical activity (or lack of it) will have to be made. Several behavioural strategies are outlined later in the chapter.

You can choose from a wide variety of foods, but have to keep within a daily allowance in the case of some foods. Some foods are prohibited, but you can eat as much as you like of others. For example, you can fill up your plate with most vegetables, which should preferably be steamed or lightly boiled. If you enjoy breakfast cereal, and choose one without added sugar, you can replace two slices of bread with 40 g (just under ½ cup) of the breakfast cereal on some mornings to vary your diet. You will obtain all the vitamins and minerals you need and do not require any supplements. As long as you keep within your allowances, you can devise your own meals to suit your circumstances and food preferences.

You can evaluate whether the programme suits you and decide if you are going to keep to it by finding out how much weight you have lost in the first four weeks. If you have lost 4 to 6 kg (9 to 13 lb.) and have not found it difficult to keep to your new eating habits, your progress is likely to be satisfactory. You will go on losing weight slowly, which is what you want.

If after four weeks you have lost less than 2 kg (4½ lb.) and find that it has been increasingly difficult to keep to your new eating habits, or if you have kept strictly to them but have lost only this amount of weight, it is worth consulting a doctor to find out the reason why you have not lost more weight. Studies have shown that the most likely reason is that your home or work environment makes it difficult to avoid the temptation to snack to overeat. In this case it may be helpful to talk to a counsellor.

One of the advantages of the programme is that within certain limits you can continue to eat the same foods as the rest of your family and your friends. This is important, because there is no reason not to continue to enjoy a social life. It is counter-productive to be a thinning, anti-social, crotchety recluse—it is better to be fat and enjoy life!

There is one proviso. The weight-reducing programme will be effective only if you really want to lose weight and are prepared to stick to the programme over a period of months. Unless you are motivated, you will find it increasingly easy, as the weeks go by, to cheat just a little—either by eating far more food than you should or by avoiding taking exercise. But many such lapses add up to a considerable excess of energy ingested and less expended, and the weight loss will cease. Persistence with the programme pays off! There is no miracle method of losing weight.

The Behavioural Aspects of Weight Reduction

Many people find that their motivation to lose weight is increased if they can share their experiences with, and obtain support from, other people who are also trying to lose weight. The support needs to extend over a period of weeks or months during the period of weight reduction. Support is also needed when they have managed to lose weight, so that they do not regain weight swiftly or insidiously. Many find it helpful to join an organization such as Weight Watchers or TOPS (Take Off Pounds Sensibly).

Membership of an organization provides a stimulus to achieve a weight loss (by a system of rewards and demerits) and provides a form of group therapy. The value of such organizations is shown by a study made in Australia in which the weight loss of women attending a hospital-based obesity clinic was compared with that of women who joined Weight Watchers. The women who had joined Weight Watchers lost more weight each week and remained at the lower weight for longer than the women who attended the obesity clinic.

It helps to keep to the weight-reducing programme if you are aware that even when you keep strictly to it, your weight may fluctuate by 1–2 kg (2–4 lb.) a week. For this reason you should not weigh yourself more than once a week, or if you can bear it, no more than once a fortnight.

....

Helpful Hints on Weight Reduction

- Try to eat your meals at approximately the same time each day. This has the psychological effect of helping you to control your feelings of hunger at times other than mealtimes.
- When you have a meal, eat slowly. When you have put food in your mouth do not add any more until your mouth is empty. If it helps, put down your knife, fork, or spoon while your mouth has food in it. And chew your food slowly so that you learn to savour the food to the fullest. Psychologists believe that eating slowly and chewing meticulously teaches you to be satisfied with less food and to enjoy the smaller quantity more. Additional dietary fibre will also help you to achieve this objective.
- Every fifteen mouthfuls, stop and put down your eating utensils for about half a minute. This helps you to enjoy the smaller amount of food more.
- Before you start eating, decide how much of which food you are going to put on your plate, and do not add more. Once you start eating it is too easy to say to yourself, 'I'll have just a little more.' You must not. A little more adds up to a lot eventually. It often helps if you put your food on a smaller plate, so that the plate looks fuller! This will help you make do with less.
- As soon as you feel full, stop eating, no matter how much is still on your plate. Indeed, it may help you always to leave some food on your plate, and so break the habit of continuing to eat until all the food on your plate has gone, whether you need it or not.
- Once you feel full or finish your meal, leave the table (if you can

do so without offending anybody). Staying at the table where there is food may break your resolve not to eat any more.

- Don't keep packets of sweets, biscuits, chocolate, or nuts in the house or office. If you get bored or unhappy you will be tempted to have a nibble. If they are not there, you can resist the temptation. If they are, you will be able to resist everything except the temptation.

- Only go shopping for food when you have eaten. If you do your own shopping, or shop for the family, you may be tempted when you see the delicious-looking foods in the shops. You can resist the temptation to buy and eat these foods if you do three simple things. First, go shopping only after you have eaten. People react less to the sight of food when they are not hungry. Second, make out a list of foods you really need before you go shopping. Stick to the list. Do not be tempted by other foods. Third, when possible, buy only foods that need more preparation than just opening the container. This will reduce the risk that you will just open a tin or a packet for a little snack.

....

Drugs in Weight Reduction

Although the use of anorectic drugs in the treatment of obesity has been enthusiastically promoted, their value is limited. Anorectic drugs reduce hunger or increase a feeling of fullness (satiety), but most obese people do not eat because of hunger. Studies have shown that patients taking a low-energy diet and anorectic medications lose more weight than those on a diet alone, but the effect diminishes or is reversed after about twelve weeks. And when the anorectic drug is stopped, weight is rapidly regained. The place of anorectic drugs in the treatment of obesity is limited. At best, they help one come to terms with the need to lose weight over a long period by boosting morale. In fact, a study of the opinions of 1,362 patients about the use of anorectic drugs showed that most preferred diet alone to diet and anorectic drugs. A minority feel that anorectic drugs help. They may take the drugs intermittently over a period of twelve to fourteen months, but no course of treatment should exceed twelve weeks. Anorectic drugs may achieve their effect by suggestion rather than by a direct action on the satiety centre in the brain. This is suggested by an investigation which demonstrated that inert injections given to a group of patients produced a greater weight loss than that achieved by most active anti-obesity drugs.

An exception to this may be a new drug, dexfenfluramine which is thought to increase the secretion of the neuro-transmitter, serotonin. Serotonin appears to play a sig-nificant role in the control of the appetite. If the level of serotonin can be raised, the desire for food is reduced and the person may become relaxed and drowsy. If the level of serotonin is lowered, the person may become irritable or anxious and hungry, especially for carbohydrate-rich snacks. Early studies using the drug show that dexfenfluramine in-creases the level of serotonin in the brain and reduces the person's urge to snack, as well as his or her appetite. It is claimed that the weight-losing action of the drug lasts for as long as a year, but in the second six months the loss of weight slows down significantly. At present the drug has been used in very few double-blind controlled studies. In one multicentre study of nearly 300 people (mainly women), half of whom were eating a restricted diet and took dexfen-fluramine and the other half of whom just ate the restricted diet and were given a placebo pill, it was found that at the end of one year the mean weight loss of the group taking dexfenfluramine was 4 kg more than the people taking the placebo, and 30 per cent of them lost more than 10 kg com-pared with 16 per cent of the people who took the placebo.

As with other drugs of this nature, about one patient in three complains of drowsiness, one in six of diarrhoea, and one in nine of a dry mouth or frequent urination. Because of this, dexfenfluramine, like other anorectic drugs, should be tried only if non-drug measures have proved inadequate.

Many other drugs have been tried. Things have not changed much since 1900 when Dr Thomas Dutton wrote in his book *Obesity*, 'quite a host of quack nostrums are advertised . . . to say the least of them, they are altogether unscientific and

in many cases positively injurious'. In Dr Dutton's day ex-
cruciating purges and strong salts were fashionable. Today,
diuretics, hormones, 'bulk fillers', and pep pills have their
advocates. Most of the drugs have been used unscientifically.
They are potentially dangerous and, except in rare circumstances, have no benefit in helping a person lose weight.
Some of them are listed below.

Short-term weight loss (up to three months)
(An average weight loss of 0.25 kg a week compared with
placebo)
   Duromine (phenteramine)
   Ponderax (fenfluoramine)
   Sanorex (madinzol)
   Tenuate (diethylproprion)

Longer-term weight loss (up to twelve months)
(An average weight loss of 2.5 kg over twelve months com-
pared with placebo)
   Adifax (dexfenfluoramine)

Drugs that have no value in aiding weight loss
   Human chorionic gonadotrophin
   Thyroid (thyroxine)—except where the person is thyroid-
     deficient
   Bulk-fillers
     Cellulone (methylcellulose)
     Starch digestion inhibitors
     Fat-absorption inhibitors

One of these, thyroid extract (thyroxine), requires special
mention as it is still prescribed by some doctors. Unless the
obese person is hypothyroid (and few are), thyroid hormone
is of no value, and should not be taken.

The problem with any slimming diet or weight-reducing
programme is that although most people achieve an initial
weight loss, few can maintain their weight within the desirable range for longer than six to twelve months. Many

glowing reports of a large weight loss achieved by this or that diet or treatment have no real validity, as the people have been followed up for too short a time. A study that covers less than twelve months presents an inaccurate success rate. In longer-term studies made over twenty years ago, it was noted that few participants lost as much as 20 kg (44 lb.) and most who did regained weight shortly after treatment ended. A decade later, a large study in Britain showed that between 10 and 40 per cent of participants had lost some weight by the end of the first year of treatment, but fewer than 10 per cent maintained the weight loss for a period of years.

Modern approaches to the problem are, first, to achieve the weight loss and, second, to maintain the lower weight by reinforcing the resolve of the person through periodic intervention in the form of supportive psychotherapy. These methods promise a more successful outcome. For example, a study of over 700 women who had reduced their weight over an average period of thirty weeks using the Weight Watchers programme, so that it fell to within the desirable range, and who continued to attend group meetings periodically, showed that fifteen months after the weight loss had been achieved only 30 per cent of the women weighed more than 10 per cent above their desirable weight.

An obese patient will achieve and maintain weight reduction only if he or she is motivated, persistent, and prepared to alter his or her life-style. If he or she is not prepared to fulfil these conditions, there is little point in persisting with a weight-reduction diet. If this occurs, the person may be prepared to visit a psychologist or a psychiatrist for assessment to determine if the habitual overeating is a maladaptation to an underlying psychological problem, such as boredom, anger, depression, or stress. A clinical psychologist or a psychiatrist may help him or her to cope with the root problem. Some obese people find it helpful to make a chart of all the food they eat during a week, noting where they were at the time, what they were doing, how they felt, and why they ate the food at that particular time. The therapist is shown the chart, and then discusses with the person how to change his or her eating behaviour.

But in the end it is up to the perseverance and motivation of the individual.

Appendix
The Foods We Eat

Solid as most of us look, over 60 per cent of our body is composed of water, two-thirds of which is held in the millions of cells which make up our body. Fat accounts for between 11 and 18 per cent of our body weight, unless we are obese, when fat makes up more. Protein, mainly in muscles, accounts for between 15 and 20 per cent of our body weight, and carbohydrate for less than 1 per cent.

The proportions of fat, protein, and carbohydrate in our body depend on the type of food and the amount of it that we eat.

Fats

Most foods that we eat contain carbohydrate, fat, and protein in varying proportions. If we eat foods that contain more fat, carbohydrate, or alcohol than we need for energy, the excess is converted into glycogen and fat. The glycogen is derived from the complex carbohydrate we eat and is stored in our liver or in the glycogen–water pool which lies between our muscle fibres (see pp. 22 and 158). The pool is not very large and when burned up releases only about 17,000 kJ (4,000 kcal) of energy. It becomes important when we need energy urgently, as it is readily obtained from this source. The excess fat in our food is stored in adipose cells in the form of triglyceride. This is now discussed further.

Different foods contain different combinations of fats, which are described, according to their chemical structure, as

- saturated fatty acids,
- mono-unsaturated fatty acids, and
- polyunsaturated fatty acids.

Saturated fatty acids are currently believed to be the 'dangerous' fats, as they are involved in causing high levels of cholesterol in our blood. Most people believe that if they stop eating fatty meat and dairy products they will reduce the amount of saturated fats that they eat. They are wrong. Cooking oils such as coconut oil and palm oil, which are used in some margarines and in some kinds of confectionery, are largely saturated. Many fast foods—cakes, biscuits, pies, pastry, and chocolate—contain a considerable quantity of saturated fat. If we want to reduce the quantity of saturated fat we eat, we have to cut down on these foods as well as eat less fatty meat and dairy products.

Mono-unsaturated fatty acids, which are mainly found in olive oil, peanuts and peanut oil, and avocados, were thought to be dangerous fats until recently. Nutritionists now believe that mono-unsaturated fats are not dangerous to our health and may reduce our blood cholesterol level to some extent.

Polyunsaturated fatty acids are found in vegetable oils, many nuts and seeds, and seafood. Polyunsaturated fats do not increase blood cholesterol, but they are fats, so any excess eaten will lead to weight gain.

Some of the fatty acids are called essential fatty acids, as they are essential to maintain the function of the cells which make up our body. Most people eating Western diets obtain enough essential fatty acids, especially linoleic acid, in their diet, and deficiency is rare.

For good health, fats (lipids) should be eaten in small quantities so that the total fat we eat constitutes less than 33 per cent of the energy we obtain from food each day. For an average man this works out at less than 70 g of fat a day, and for an average woman less than 50 g a day.

When we eat foods containing animal or vegetable fats, we are eating, in chemical terms, cholesterol and fatty acid esters of glycerol and alcohol. The fatty acid esters of glycerol occur in our food as mixed triglycerides.

Cholesterol is absorbed from food directly while the mixed tri-glycerides are broken down in the gut into fatty acids, monogly-cerides, and glycerol. In the cells lining the gut these fatty acids, monoglycerides, and glycerol are reconverted into triglycerides and are absorbed into the blood. In the blood, cholesterol and the trigly-cerides combine with protein to form lipoproteins which transport them around the body. An average adult person living in Britain or the USA eats 120 g of triglycerides and 0.5 g of cholesterol each day.

There are four classes of lipoprotein: chylomicrons, very low density lipoprotein (VLDL), low density lipoprotein (LDL), and high density lipoprotein (HDL).

The chylomicrons, which carry triglycerides to the liver, consist mainly of ingested triglycerides with a small amount of cholesterol. Chylomicrons are formed immediately after a meal and circulate for about twelve hours, after which they are metabolized. VLDL mainly carries triglyceride with a small amount of cholesterol around the body where some is released into the blood and some is released in the liver, but most is taken to the adipose tissue for storage. When energy is needed, the triglycerides are broken down into free fatty acids, and the energy obtained is released into the blood.

HDL and LDL are formed in the liver from VLDL and, as they enter the blood, they carry cholesterol with a small amount of triglyceride to the tissues. LDL carries cholesterol to the liver and the tissues, while HDL carries cholesterol from the tissues to the liver, where it is broken down. The absolute level of cholesterol and the relative levels of HDL and LDL in our blood are a measure of the chance that we will have a heart attack.

Cholesterol is not just a 'bad' substance which increases the chance of a heart attack. Most cholesterol is made in the liver, and the cholesterol from food is added to the total. Cholesterol has essential functions in the body. It becomes bad only when its level in the blood and tissues is too high. Cholesterol is essential for the function of body cells; it makes the sheaths of nerve fibres; and it is the starting-point of steroid hormones.

Adipose tissue is composed of fat cells, which make up about four-fifths of its volume, and water which makes up one-fifth, with a trace of protein. When we need energy over a period of time, for example during a famine, energy is released from the adipose tissue and we become thinner and thinner.

For people living in places where starvation often occurs, it makes sense to have extra fat stored in the body, but for most of us the extra fat is not needed except to give our bodies a rounded contour. In fact, excess fat, which causes obesity, may be a health risk. Heart attacks are more likely to occur if most of the fat is deposited around the belly, giving the person an apple shape, rather than around the hips which gives the person a pear shape.

Proteins

Proteins are basic chemical units of the body which are essential for nutrition, growth, and repair. They make up about 15 per cent of our body mass. All our body cells contain proteins, but most of the proteins in our body are in our muscles, our heart, liver, kidneys, and blood cells.

Proteins are complex substances made up of simpler substances called amino acids. Various combinations of the amino acids (there are twenty-three of them) make up proteins. Most proteins contain between fifty and 1,000 molecules of combinations of amino acids strung out on a long chain, like a necklace. Every species of plant and animal has characteristic proteins.

Plants synthesize their proteins from inorganic substances—carbon, nitrogen, oxygen, and hydrogen—under the influence of sunlight. Animals are unable to synthesize proteins and have to obtain their protein by eating plants or other animals. Animals can convert fifteen of the twenty-three amino acids into other amino acid combinations in the liver, but there are eight amino acids which animals cannot make for themselves and must obtain from their food. These amino acids are called essential amino acids because without them protein-deficiency diseases may result.

When we eat food containing protein it is broken down into its constituent amino acids in the gut, and these are absorbed into our body to be used to replace decaying protein or to be reconstituted into new proteins in the liver.

The greater the turnover of the body tissues, the greater is the need for protein. In infancy and childhood, for example, more protein is needed because the body is growing rapidly. If the child is unable to obtain sufficient protein, mental dullness and protein-deficiency diseases may result. In the poor countries of the world and among the most deprived groups of some rich countries, many infants and young children fail to obtain sufficient protein and energy from the inadequate diet that they eat. In addition, protein deficiency may affect the cells that line the gut so that the limited food available is less well absorbed. This may result in protein-energy deficiency. Children who have protein-energy deficiency become thin, wasted, and may develop pot-bellies. They often have diarrhoea, because their resistance to infection is reduced. Such images have often appeared on our television screens. At least 100 million children under the age of 5 in the developing countries have protein-energy deficiency and many die each year.

The average daily need of protein for an adult is between 45 and 55 g a day. Most of us in Western countries obtain between 60 and 70 g a day from the food we eat, mainly from meat, eggs, and dairy products, so that protein deficiency rarely occurs. However, animal products are expensive, and most of the world's inhabitants obtain their protein from cereals, grains, and vegetables. Most people living in the developing countries eat little meat, but they eat a variety of cereals and vegetables so that they obtain all the protein they need, provided they survive childhood when, as mentioned, protein-energy deficiency is common.

Women who are pregnant or who are breast-feeding need an extra 10 g or so of protein a day, which they can obtain by drinking an extra 250 ml of milk or eating an extra cheese sandwich. Some athletes believe that they should eat extra protein or take protein powders for perfect performance. There is no benefit in choosing either of these: if the athlete is hungry he or she will obtain the extra energy and all the protein needed from an extra helping of food!

The protein we eat provides the materials for tissue growth and repair, and a quantity of energy is released when protein is broken down into its amino acids: 1 g of protein releases about 19 kJ (4.5 kcal) of energy. This energy is not important to the body unless the person has been starving for some time and has burned up all the body fat. If this occurs, protein in muscles may be burned up to provide energy needed for survival. This results in muscle-wasting and weakness.

There may be a problem among people who eat little or no animal foods (for example vegetarians). Cereal, grain, and vegetable protein usually lack one or more of the essential amino acids, so that to maintain good health you should eat a mixed diet of cereals, vegetables, and pulses, which will provide all the essential amino acids.

Carbohydrates

We obtain most of the energy our body needs from the carbohydrates we eat. Carbohydrates are synthesized by plants from carbon dioxide in the air and water, under the influence of sunlight. There are two main classes of carbohydrate—complex carbohydrates and simple carbohydrates. Complex carbohydrates (starches and glycogen) are made up of thousands of units of glucose. Simple carbohydrates include sucrose (cane sugar), maltose, glucose, lactose (milk sugar), and fructose (fruit sugar).

Complex carbohydrates occur in all cereal and grain foods and in foods based on cereals and grains, such as bread, pasta, and rice. Complex carbohydrates are also found in legumes such as peas, beans, and lentils, and in vegetables. Most plant foods contain some protein and varying quantities of fat, as well as complex carbohydrate.

When a food containing complex carbohydrate is eaten, the starch is broken down into glucose and fructose, as this is the only way in which carbohydrates can be absorbed by the body.

The process begins in the mouth when an enzyme in saliva begins to break down the carbohydrate. After swallowing, the food mass reaches the stomach where hydrochloric acid mixes with it and acts on the protein in the food. The stomach also acts as a reservoir for food, squirting out small amounts into the intestines at intervals.

Complex carbohydrates are mainly digested in the small intestine where the starch is acted on by an enzyme (amylase) to convert it into maltose and sucrose. Maltose and sucrose are absorbed into the lining cells of the gut and are further simplified, being converted into glucose. Glucose enters the bloodstream and the level of glucose rises. This induces the pancreatic gland to secrete insulin into the blood which acts on glucose and helps to convert it into the storage carbohydrate, glycogen, which is deposited in the liver and in the muscles. When the liver and muscle stores (the glycogen–water pool) are full, any extra glucose is converted into fat. This adds to fat stores, but to a lesser extent than the fat released from fatty foods.

The liver glycogen helps to keep the level of glucose in the blood in the normal range. If the level falls, glycogen is converted into glucose which enters the blood; if the level of glucose rises, as after a meal, insulin is released which facilitates the conversion of glucose into glycogen.

Glucose is of supreme importance in providing energy to maintain the functions of the body and, except in extreme starvation, is the only fuel that the brain can use.

As mentioned, most foods consist of a mixture of varying proportions of carbohydrate, fat, and protein. The digestion of simple carbohydrate is quite fast; complex carbohydrates take longer to digest, in part because they contain non-starch polysaccharide or dietary fibre (which is discussed on pages 58–68). Foods made up largely of protein and fat take still longer to digest, and remain longer in the stomach, which is one reason why you feel full after eating a meal with a high proportion of fat.

As far as our health is concerned, our diet should contain between 45 and 50 per cent complex carbohydrate and no more than 5 to 10 per cent sugar. These proportions permits us to fill our glycogen stores and have a good amount left over for our body's needs, including exercise.

Vitamins

These are discussed in Chapter 11.

Selected Minerals

In this section only selected minerals are discussed. (Further details can be found in *Dietary Reference Values for Food Energy and Nutrients for the United Kingdom* (HMSO, 1991)). The two minerals we are most likely to be deficient in, iron and calcium, have been discussed in Chapter 12. Other minerals a deficiency or excess of which may cause illness are sodium, potassium, magnesium, and zinc.

Sodium

Sodium is the main constituent of salt. Most of us eat about ten to twenty times as much salt each day as we need. We obtain this from highly salted processed and fast foods, and from adding salt to our cooking and to cooked food. Many of us sprinkle salt on our food without even tasting it. The reason is that we like the taste of salted foods, and find food without salt tasteless. The taste for salt is not inborn but learned, as is shown by the fact that many primitive peoples eat diets that contain little salt.

Many people believe that additional salt is needed if we undertake vigorous exercise in hot weather. Sweat tastes salty, so we think we must be losing a considerable amount of salt when we sweat. It is true that we do lose some salt in our sweat, but we lose much more water, which should be replaced before we think of eating a salty food. It is also believed that muscle cramps are due to salt loss. This is untrue.

Much of the salt we eat is hidden in foods, for example a bowl of cornflakes contains nearly three times as much salt as a packet of potato crisps.

There is now some evidence that too much salt in the diet is a factor in high blood pressure which may lead to a stroke. If you want to reduce your salt intake, start by ceasing to sprinkle salt on your food. Follow this by using about three-quarters as much salt in cooking. If you want to add flavour to cooking, use herbs and spices.

It takes time for our taste buds to recover from years of habituation to salt. After two weeks, we will cease to want more salt; after four weeks we will be able to accept less salty foods; after twelve weeks we may prefer unsalted foods.

Potassium

It has been said, 'Look after the sodium and the potassium will look after itself.' Potassium balances the effects of sodium in the body cells and tissues. Most of the body's potassium is inside body cells and most sodium is outside the cells, in the spaces between the cells and in the blood. The distribution of sodium and potassium is regulated by substances produced in the kidneys, usually with great precision.

Potassium is essential for the proper transmission of nerve impulses and for the functioning of the heart. A deficiency of potassium is likely only if the person has prolonged diarrhoea and vomiting, and among some people with anorexia nervosa or bulimia, who starve themselves, abuse laxatives, or induce vomiting frequently. Potassium deficiency may also occur if a person is prescribed diuretics to control his or her high blood pressure. This is the reason why doctors give potassium tablets to patients taking these drugs.

Most people obtain all the potassium they need from the food they eat. Many vegetables and fruits are rich in potassium. If we eat large amounts of processed foods, which are often rich in sodium, we may become potassium deficient unless we vary our diet to include vegetables and fruit.

Magnesium

Magnesium is involved with calcium in the growth and maintenance of bone, and the maintenance of nerve and muscle function. Most people obtain all the magnesium they need from the food they eat. Magnesium is obtained from cereals, meats, and green vegetables.

An adult needs about 250 mg a day, and the food we eat easily supplies this amount for most people. A few people, particularly chronic alcoholics, those who have prolonged diarrhoea and vomiting, and those who are starving may become magnesium deficient. When this occurs the muscles become weak and the heart-beat may become irregular.

Zinc

Zinc is an essential component of many enzymes which keep our body functioning, particularly in the metabolism of proteins, carbohydrates, and fats. Zinc is obtained mainly from animal foods (oysters are particularly rich in zinc). Absorption of zinc is diminished if there is much phytate in the food. Phytate is found in wholegrain cereal products, so if we eat large amounts of unprocessed bran (more than two tablespoonfuls a day) we may become deficient in zinc. In some developing countries, children whose diet consists mainly of wholegrain foods may develop zinc deficiency. This may lead to growth retardation, poor sexual development, and slow healing of skin wounds. In some adult men in these countries, zinc deficiency may cause a decrease in sperm production.

In Western countries people are unlikely to become zinc deficient unless they drink a good deal of alcohol or eat a lot of unprocessed bran.

Some health fanatics claim that if you take extra zinc you will grow taller, your skin will become unmarked and perfect, and your sexual performance will be enhanced. They claim to be able to detect zinc deficiency by doing a hair analysis. Both of these claims are false. You can detect zinc deficiency only by measuring its level in a blood sample. Extra zinc does none of the things claimed for it.

Water and Electrolytes

Even if all flesh is as grass, the human body is mostly water. Sixty per cent of its weight is water. This means that if you weigh 60 kg, the water in your body will measure 36 l and weigh 36 kg. Two-thirds of this water is within the millions of cells that make up your body tissues. The remaining third lies outside the cells, making up the fluids of your blood and your lymph, and lying in the narrow spaces between cells. The water in your body is not pure. It contains quantities of sodium, potassium, magnesium, and calcium, usually combined with chloride, which gives it a resemblance to sea water (and perhaps hints at our maritime origins). When these minerals are dissolved in water they are called electrolytes, and there is a constant movement of electrolytes between the water within the cells and that between the cells. The transfer of the electrolytes is essential for the processes that keep the cells alive and functioning, and with each movement of sodium into the cells, or of potassium out of the cells, energy is used.

Salt, in the form of sodium chloride, is the most important electrolyte, as has been mentioned earlier, we have either always needed or been conditioned to eat salt. The singular importance of salt as part of the diet is demonstrated by the fact that for centuries trade in salt was more important than trade in any other commodity. Salt is not only needed to maintain the composition of body water, but is an excellent food preservative. In general, most people eat as much salt as they need to maintain the electrolyte balance of their body fluids, but habit plays a part. Some primitive groups eat very little salt and seem to be healthy. In contrast, many Western people eat more salt than they need because custom has habituated the taste buds in their tongue to require salty foods. There is some evidence that an addiction to salt (in temperate climates, at least) may be damaging to health. It has been observed that people living in northern Japan eat twice as much salt as those living in southern Japan. The northern Japanese have a much greater chance of developing high blood pressure and of dying from strokes. This is not to suggest that excessive salt eaten over the years causes high blood pressure, but it may be a factor. It would be wise to abstain from eating too much salt.

The water that makes up the largest proportion of our body comes from the fluid we drink, from the water content of the food we eat, and from the burning up or oxidation of that food in our body. Each gram of starch, when it is used up, releases about 0.6 g of water; each gram of protein utilized releases about 0.4 g of water; and each gram of fat burned up yields just under 1 g of water. Throughout the day we lose fluid from the body. It is lost in the urine, in the sweat, in the air we breathe out, and in the fluids we secrete into the gut.

In this way a fluid balance is established: the amount of fluid taken into our body in food and drink, or created by burning up food in our body, is balanced by the amount of fluid we lose. If the balance is upset and we lose more fluid than we obtain, we become dehydrated. In severe cases of dehydration the eyes become sunken, the skin and tongue are dry, the lips are cracked and hard, and the skin loses its elasticity. If you pinch the skin of a dehydrated person it will stand up away from the underlying tissue. Dehydration may occur during fever, because the body tries to keep the temperature down by increased evaporation of fluid from the skin and lungs. It occurs in cholera and other diseases that cause severe diarrhoea because of the fluid taken from the body by the inflamed cells that line the gut. Dehydration occurs in hot climates if we do not drink enough fluids. In all cases of dehydration, sodium chloride is lost with the water, so we become deficient both in water and in electrolytes.

If the electrolyte and water balance is changed in the opposite direction, we retain more fluid in the body than we lose. When the body water is increased by 10 per cent or more (that is, by about 3 l in an average person) the fluid becomes obvious, and a condition called oedema results. The limbs become swollen, especially around the lower legs and ankles, and if you press your thumb into the swollen area and keep it pressed for about half a minute, a pit will appear and will remain for a while after your thumb has been removed.

Energy

A major function of the food we eat is to provide energy so that our body can function properly. The amount of energy we require each day depends on our age, our body size, the type of work we do, and our leisure activities. It is obvious that a 75-year-old woman weighing 50 kg who spends most of her time sitting watching television or knitting requires less energy than a 25-year-old lumberjack weighing 80 kg.

During a twenty-four-hour period, we spend about eight hours in bed or sitting. During this time energy is needed for the unconscious activities of our body. It is needed to enable the heart to beat seventy times a minute, 4,200 times an hour, 100,800 times a day, forcing blood round the body with each beat. Energy is needed to make our muscles contract so that we may breathe, and to keep the other muscles supple and ready for fight or flight. Energy is needed to help us digest the food we have eaten. Energy is needed to maintain all these body functions day in, day out. The energy needed for these activities is defined by physiologists as the energy expended by a person who is relaxed and comfortable in a warm environment, soon after waking up and about twelve hours after last eating a meal. This is called the resting or basal metabolic rate.

We spend an average of five and a half hours a day each week at work, whether outside our home in employment or in our home in unpaid housework. The amount of energy required will depend on the type of work we do, but today, with labour-saving machines and devices, less heavy manual work is being undertaken. Machines, not men, dig ditches.

We spend the rest of the twenty-four hours in leisure activities, including travelling to work. Leisure activities vary depending on personal preference. Some people expend a great deal of energy in one leisure activity, for example playing squash or running. Much less energy is expended by the person who goes to the cinema or watches television.

TABLE I. *Energy requirements* (per day)

Age	Average weight (kg)	Energy (kJ/kcal)
Children		
1–3	13.4	5,200 (1,240)
4–6	18.0	7,190 (1,720)
7–9	27.0	8,400 (2,000)
Men		
11–14	45.0	9,250 (2,220)
15–18	65.0	11,500 (2,755)
19–29	70.0	12,500 (3,000)
30–59	75.0	12,240 (2,900)
60–75	72.0	9,000 (2,200)
Women		
11–14	40.0	7,920 (1,845)
15–18	54.0	8,830 (2,110)
19–29	60.0	9,660 (2,300)
30–59	62.0	10,000 (2,400)
60–75	63.0	8,000 (1,900)
Pregnant women		+950 (230)

It is possible to make calculations to determine how much energy is needed each day for these activities. It will vary, of course, depending on age, weight, and activity level.

In infancy, childhood, and adolescence more energy is needed for the growth of the body; in contrast, in old age less energy is needed as the resting metabolic rate drops slightly and the person usually becomes less active.

Any energy that is in excess of the energy needed for the resting metabolic rate, the digestion of food, and work and leisure activities is converted in the body and added to the fat stores.

Exact calculations of the amount of energy expended each day by an individual can be made from complicated tables but, except for research purposes, they are not practical. Two simplified tables are given here to give you an idea of energy expenditure. The first table shows the average energy requirements of people of different ages and body weights.

The second table shows the energy expenditure of two people—a man between the age of 20 and 35 who weighs 75 kg and a woman in the same age range who weighs 60 kg.

TABLE 2. *Energy expenditure* (per day)

Activity	Hours	Activity (kJ/kcal)		
		Light	Moderate	Heavy
Man aged 20–35, weighing 75 kg				
In bed	8	2,400 (580)	2,400 (580)	2,400 (580)
At work	5.5	2,850 (680)	4,500 (1,070)	5,020 (1,200)
Leisure activity	10.5	4,800 (1,140)	5,430 (1,300)	6,000 (1,430)
Average daily energy expenditure		10,050 (2,390)	12,240 (2,910)	13,420 (3,195)
Woman aged 20–35, weighing 60 kg				
In bed	8	1,880 (450)	1,880 (450)	1,880 (450)
At work	5.5	2,850 (680)	3,680 (877)	3,850 (917)
Leisure activity	10.5	3,700 (880)	4,180 (1,000)	4,680 (1,450)
Average daily energy expenditure		8,430 (2,007)	9,660 (2,300)	10,410 (2,500)

Source: Calculations derived from data in *Dietary Reference Values for Food Energy and Nutrients for the United Kingdom* (HMSO, 1991) and *Energy and Protein Requirements* (Tech. Rep. Series 724, WHO).

The calculations in this table assume that the person spends eight hours in bed, has a working week of five days, works for seven and a half hours each day, and spends the rest of the time in different types of leisure activity. The type of work and the leisure activities can be graded as light, moderate, or heavy.

Light activity (averaged out) includes watching television, reading, sewing, ironing, washing dishes, general office or laboratory work. Moderate activity includes making beds, cleaning the house, painting, decorating, light manufacturing, carpentry, bricklaying, motor-vehicle repairing, playing golf or cricket. Heavy activity includes climbing stairs, chopping wood, heavy gardening, labouring, road construction, digging, felling trees, dancing, jogging, football, tennis, energetic swimming, cycling.

The table shows how much energy an average person expends in these activities.

Glossary

Adipose tissue The tissues of the body that contain large numbers of fat cells. The composition of adipose tissue is 80 per cent fat, 2 per cent protein, and the remainder is water. Because of the high proportion of fat, adipose tissue is often called fatty tissue.

Amino acids The 20 chemical substances that combine, in an almost infinite number of ways, to produce protein.

Aneurism A weakened, bulging area usually in the wall of the main artery of the body (the aorta).

Appetite The sensation that makes you want to eat a particular food. Often confused with hunger.

Body mass index (BMI) A measure to determine if a person is of normal weight, underweight, or overweight.

Carbohydrates The class of nutrients made up of starches and sugars. See pp. 177–9 for further details.

Defecate To open the bowels or pass a stool.

Electrolytes See p. 180 for definition.

Energy Energy is needed for the body to function. It is measured in joules (kilojoules and megajoules) or in calories (kilocalories or kcal). To convert calories into joules multiply by 4.2.

Enzymes Chemical substances produced in the body which are essential to cause chemical transformation of material in plants and animals.

FAO The United Nations Food and Agricultural Organization.

Fibre The part of the plant that is not digested by humans. This includes the plant cell wall (lignin) and parts of the cell (some polysaccharides).

Foetus The growing baby while still in its mother's uterus.

Glycogen The form in which excess carbohydrate is stored in the body.

Gram A measure of weight, equivalent to ½8th of an ounce. Usually abbreviated to g.

Hunger The sensation that makes you want to eat. Often confused with appetite.

Incidence The number of cases in a given community occurring (or being detected) in a specific period, usually one year.

Lipids The biochemical term for fats (see pp. 174–5 for full discussion).

Nutrition The action or process of receiving substances that aid tissue growth and repair, thus promoting the well-being of the body.

Oedema The swelling of tissues owing to fluid lying in the spaces between the cells that make up the tissue.

Parboiled The rice (still in the husk) is steamed before it is milled. This 'fixes' thiamin to the grain and milling does not remove it.

Polyunsaturated fatty acids See p. 174.

Prevalence The number of cases in a given community, usually expressed as the number per every 1,000 population.

Protein See pp. 175–7 for definition.

Resting (basal) metabolic rate (RMR) The energy expended by a person for the vital unconscious processes of the body, which keep it running. These include: heat production, digestion, breathing, and the work of the heart to keep the blood circulating.

Saturated fatty acids See p. 173.

Triglycerides A substance made up of three fatty acids linked and held by glycerol (monoglycerides have only one fatty acid linked with glycerol).

Index

osteoporosis 149–52
  causes of 148, 149
  costs of 150
  prevention of, 150–2

parathyroid hormone 144
pellagra 115–16
physical activity:
  benefits of 9
  changes in past years 7–8
  choices in 10–11
  lack of 86
  principles of 10
  sport 11
  types of: aerobic 9; anaerobic 10;
    isometric 10
  weight loss and 160
phytate 130, 135
plaque (in arteries) 82
potassium 179
proteins 175–7
  daily requirement 176

resting metabolic rate 22
rice 110
rickets 101–3
  cure of 104
  prevention of 102, 103

salt 181
scurvy 118–19
skin fold thickness 26
sloth 8, 11
  coronary heart disease and 86
smoking 152
sodium 178
starch 36
starvation 29, 159
sugar 39, 46–8
  benefits of 50
  consumption of 46–8
  energy in diet from 48–9
  harm from eating 50–4
  health problems 50
  'hidden' 48
  obesity and 56
sweet tooth 49

thiamin 111
tooth, sweet 49

triglycerides 81

varicose veins 63
vegans 96, 141
very low density lipoprotein (VLDL)
  81
vitamins:
  discovery of 94–5
  myths about 96–7
vitamin A 20, 97–100
  benefits of 97–8
  blindness and 97–8
  cancer and 99
  dangers of 100
  heart disease and 98
  liver damage and 99
  sources of 99
vitamin B group 110–19
  B$_{12}$ 138, 139, 141
  niacin 20, 116, 117
  thiamine 110–17
  sources of 117
vitamin C (ascorbic acid) 118–26,
  137
  common cold and 123–5
  scurvy and 118–19
  sources of 121
vitamin D 100–5, 142–4
  excess of, dangers 104
  rickets and 101
  sources of 104
vitamin E 20, 105–10
  heart disease, in 109
  prematurity, in 107
  skin conditions, in 108
vitamin K 96

water, body content of 180–1
weight:
  concern about 5, 6
  reducing programmes:
    behavioural aspects of 166;
    drugs in 168–70; hints for 167;
    physical activity during 160;
    principles of 156–9, 162–3;
    programme for 158, 159, 160–2,
    164–5; strategies for 159

zinc 67, 127, 180

OXFORD

MORE OXFORD PAPERBACKS

This book is just one of nearly 1000 Oxford Paperbacks currently in print. If you would like details of other Oxford Paperbacks, including titles in the World's Classics, Oxford Reference, Oxford Books, OPUS, Past Masters, Oxford Authors, and Oxford Shakespeare series, please write to:

UK and Europe: Oxford Paperbacks Publicity Manager, Arts and Reference Publicity Department, Oxford University Press, Walton Street, Oxford OX2 6DP.

Customers in UK and Europe will find Oxford Paperbacks available in all good bookshops. But in case of difficulty please send orders to the Cash-with-Order Department, Oxford University Press Distribution Services, Saxon Way West, Corby, Northants NN18 9ES. Tel: 0536 741519; Fax: 0536 746337. Please send a cheque for the total cost of the books, plus £1.75 postage and packing for orders under £20; £2.75 for orders over £20. Customers outside the UK should add 10% of the cost of the books for postage and packing.

USA: Oxford Paperbacks Marketing Manager, Oxford University Press, Inc., 200 Madison Avenue, New York, N.Y. 10016.

Canada: Trade Department, Oxford University Press, 70 Wynford Drive, Don Mills, Ontario M3C 1J9.

Australia: Trade Marketing Manager, Oxford University Press, G.P.O. Box 2784Y, Melbourne 3001, Victoria.

South Africa: Oxford University Press, P.O. Box 1141, Cape Town 8000.

WOMEN'S STUDIES FROM
OXFORD PAPERBACKS

Ranging from the *A–Z of Women's Health* to *Wayward Women: A Guide to Women Travellers*, Oxford Paperbacks cover a wide variety of social, medical, historical, and literary topics of particular interest to women.

DESTINED TO BE WIVES
The Sisters of Beatrice Webb
Barbara Caine

Drawing on their letters and diaries, Barbara Caine's fascinating account of the lives of Beatrice Webb and her sisters, the Potters, presents a vivid picture of the extraordinary conflicts and tragedies taking place behind the respectable façade which has traditionally characterized Victorian and Edwardian family life.

The tensions and pressures of family life, particularly for women; the suicide of one sister; the death of another, probably as a result of taking cocaine after a family breakdown; the shock felt by the older sisters at the promiscuity of their younger sister after the death of her husband are all vividly recounted. In all the crises they faced, the sisters formed the main network of support for each other, recognizing that the 'sisterhood' provided the only security in a society which made women subordinate to men, socially, legally, and economically.

Other women's studies titles:

A–Z of Women's Health   Derek Llewellyn-Jones
'Victorian Sex Goddess': Lady Colin Campbell and the Sensational Divorce Case of 1886   G. H. Fleming
Wayward Women: A Guide to Women Travellers
Jane Robinson
Catherine the Great: Life and Legend   John T. Alexander

POLITICS IN OXFORD PAPERBACKS

Oxford Paperbacks offers incisive and provocative studies of the political ideologies and institutions that have shaped the modern world since 1945.

GOD SAVE ULSTER!

The Religion and Politics of Paisleyism

Steve Bruce

Ian Paisley is the only modern Western leader to have founded his own Church and political party, and his enduring popularity and success mirror the complicated issues which continue to plague Northern Ireland. This book is the first serious analysis of his religious and political careers and a unique insight into Unionist politics and religion in Northern Ireland today.

Since it was founded in 1951, the Free Presbyterian Church of Ulster has grown steadily; it now comprises some 14,000 members in fifty congregations in Ulster and ten branches overseas. The Democratic Unionist Party, formed in 1971, now speaks for about half of the Unionist voters in Northern Ireland, and the personal standing of the man who leads both these movements was confirmed in 1979 when Ian R. K. Paisley received more votes than any other member of the European Parliament. While not neglecting Paisley's 'charismatic' qualities, Steve Bruce argues that the key to his success has been his ability to embody and represent traditional evangelical Protestantism and traditional Ulster Unionism.

'original and profound . . . I cannot praise this book too highly.' Bernard Crick, *New Society*

Also in Oxford Paperbacks:

Freedom Under Thatcher   Keith Ewing and Conor Gearty
Strong Leadership   Graham Little
The Thatcher Effect   Dennis Kavanagh and Anthony Seldon

SCIENCE IN OXFORD PAPERBACKS

Oxford Paperbacks' expanding science and mathematics list offers a range of books across the scientific spectrum by men and women at the forefront of their fields, including Richard Dawkins, Martin Gardner, James Lovelock, Raymond Smullyan, and Nobel Prize winners Peter Medawar and Gerald Edelman.

THE SELFISH GENE

Second Edition

Richard Dawkins

Our genes made us. We animals exist for their preservation and are nothing more than their throwaway survival machines. The world of the selfish gene is one of savage competition, ruthless exploitation, and deceit. But what of the acts of apparent altruism found in nature—the bees who commit suicide when they sting to protect the hive, or the birds who risk their lives to warn the flock of an approaching hawk? Do they contravene the fundamental law of gene selfishness? By no means: Dawkins shows that the selfish gene is also the subtle gene. And he holds out the hope that our species—alone on earth—has the power to rebel against the designs of the selfish gene. This book is a call to arms. It is both manual and manifesto, and it grips like a thriller.

The Selfish Gene, Richard Dawkins's brilliant first book and still his most famous, is an international bestseller in thirteen languages. For this greatly expanded edition, endnotes have been added, giving fascinating reflections on the original text, and there are two major new chapters.

'learned, witty, and very well written . . . exhilaratingly good.' Sir Peter Medawar, *Spectator*

'Who should read this book? Everyone interested in the universe and their place in it.' Jeffrey R. Baylis, *Animal Behaviour*

'the sort of popular science writing that makes the reader feel like a genius' *New York Times*

Also in Oxford Paperbacks:

The Extended Phenotype   Richard Dawkins
The Ages of Gaia   James Lovelock
The Unheeded Cry   Bernard E. Rollin

LAW FROM OXFORD PAPERBACKS

Oxford Paperbacks's law list ranges from introductions to the English legal system to reference books and in-depth studies of contemporary legal issues.

INTRODUCTION TO ENGLISH LAW
Tenth Edition

William Geldart
Edited by D. C. M. Yardley

'Geldart' has over the years established itself as a standard account of English law, expounding the body of modern law as set in its historical context. Regularly updated since its first publication, it remains indispensable to student and layman alike as a concise, reliable guide.

Since publication of the ninth edition in 1984 there have been important court decisions and a great deal of relevant new legislation. D. C. M. Yardley, Chairman of the Commission for Local Administration in England, has taken account of all these developments and the result has been a considerable rewriting of several parts of the book. These include the sections dealing with the contractual liability of minors, the abolition of the concept of illegitimacy, the liability of a trade union in tort for inducing a person to break his/her contract of employment, the new public order offences, and the intent necessary for a conviction of murder.

Other law titles:

Freedom Under Thatcher: Civil Liberties in Modern Britain
Keith Ewing and Conor Gearty
Doing the Business Dick Hobbs
Judges David Pannick
Law and Modern Society P. S. Atiyah

PHILOSOPHY IN OXFORD PAPERBACKS

Ranging from authoritative introductions in the Past Masters and OPUS series to in-depth studies of classical and modern thought, the Oxford Paperbacks' philosophy list is one of the most provocative and challenging available.

THE GREAT PHILOSOPHERS
Bryan Magee

Beginning with the death of Socrates in 399, and following the story through the centuries to recent figures such as Bertrand Russell and Wittgenstein, Bryan Magee and fifteen contemporary writers and philosophers provide an accessible and exciting introduction to Western philosophy and its greatest thinkers.

Bryan Magee in conversation with:

A. J. Ayer	John Passmore
Michael Ayers	Anthony Quinton
Miles Burnyeat	John Searle
Frederick Copleston	Peter Singer
Hubert Dreyfus	J. P. Stern
Anthony Kenny	Geoffrey Warnock
Sidney Morgenbesser	Bernard Williams
Martha Nussbaum	

'Magee is to be congratulated . . . anyone who sees the programmes or reads the book will be left in no danger of believing philosophical thinking is unpractical and uninteresting.' Ronald Hayman, *Times Educational Supplement*

'one of the liveliest, fast-paced introductions to philosophy, ancient and modern that one could wish for' *Universe*

Also by Bryan Magee in Oxford Paperbacks:

Men of Ideas
Aspects of Wagner 2/e

MEDICINE IN OXFORD PAPERBACKS

Oxford Paperbacks offers an increasing list of medical studies and reference books of interest to the specialist and general reader alike, including The Facts series, authoritative and practical guides to a wide range of common diseases and conditions.

CONCISE MEDICAL DICTIONARY
Third Edition

Written without the use of unnecessary technical jargon, this illustrated medical dictionary will be welcomed as a home reference, as well as an indispensible aid for all those working in the medical profession.

Nearly 10,000 important terms and concepts are explained, including all the major medical and surgical specialities, such as gynaecology and obstetrics, paediatrics, dermatology, neurology, cardiology, and tropical medicine. This third edition contains much new material on pre-natal diagnosis, infertility treatment, nuclear medicine, community health, and immunology. Terms relating to advances in molecular biology and genetic engineering have been added, and recently developed drugs in clinical use are included. A feature of the dictionary is its unusually full coverage of the fields of community health, psychology, and psychiatry.

Each entry contains a straightforward definition, followed by a more detailed description, while an extensive crossreference system provides the reader with a comprehensive view of a particular subject.

Also in Oxford Paperbacks:

Drugs and Medicine   Roderick Cawson and Roy Spector
Travellers' Health: How to Stay Healthy Abroad 2/e
Richard Dawood
I'm a Health Freak Too!
Aidan Macfarlane and Ann McPherson
Problem Drinking   Nick Heather and Ian Robertson

RELIGION AND THEOLOGY FROM
OXFORD PAPERBACKS

The Oxford Paperbacks's religion and theology list offers the most balanced and authoritative coverage of the history, institutions, and leading figures of the Christian churches, as well as providing in-depth studies of the world's most important religions.

MICHAEL RAMSEY
A Life

Owen Chadwick

Lord Ramsey of Canterbury, Archbishop of Canterbury from 1961 to 1974, and one of the best-loved and most influential churchmen of this century, died on 23 April 1988.

Drawing on Dr Ramsey's private papers and free access to the Lambeth Palace archive, Owen Chadwick's biography is a masterly account of Ramsey's life and works. He became Archbishop of Canterbury as Britain entered an unsettled age. At home he campaigned politically against racialism and determined to secure justice and equality for immigrants. In Parliament he helped to abolish capital punishment and to relax the laws relating to homosexuality. Abroad he was a stern opponent of apartheid, both in South Africa and Rhodesia. In Christendom at large he promoted a new spirit of brotherhood among the churches, and benefited from the ecumenism of Popes John XXIII and Paul VI, and the leaders of the Orthodox Churches of Eastern Europe.

Dr Ramsey emerges from this book as a person of much prayer and rock-like conviction, who in an age of shaken belief and pessimism was an anchor of faith and hope.

Other religion and theology titles:

John Henry Newman: A Biography   Ian Ke
John Calvin   William Bouwsma
A History of Heresy   David Christie-Murra
The Wisdom of the Saints   Jill Haak Adels

OXFORD REFERENCE

Oxford is famous for its superb range of dictionaries and reference books. The Oxford Reference series offers the most up-to-date and comprehensive paperbacks at the most competitive prices, across a broad spectrum of subjects.

THE CONCISE OXFORD COMPANION
TO ENGLISH LITERATURE

Edited by Margaret Drabble and Jenny Stringer

Based on the immensely popular fifth edition of the *Oxford Companion to English Literature* this is an indispensable, compact guide to the central matter of English literature.

There are more than 5,000 entries on the lives and works of authors, poets, playwrights, essayists, philosophers, and historians; plot summaries of novels and plays; literary movements; fictional characters; legends; theatres; periodicals; and much more.

The book's sharpened focus on the English literature of the British Isles makes it especially convenient to use, but there is still generous coverage of the literature of other countries and of other disciplines which have influenced or been influenced by English literature.

From reviews of *The Oxford Companion to English Literature Fifth Edition:*

'a book which one turns to with constant pleasure . . . a book with much style and little prejudice' Iain Gilchrist, *TLS*

'it is quite difficult to imagine, in this genre, a more useful publication' Frank Kermode, *London Review of Books*

'incarnates a living sense of tradition . . . sensitive not to fashion merely but to the spirit of the age' Christopher Ricks, *Sunday Times*

Also available in Oxford Reference:

The Concise Oxford Dictionary of Art and Artists
edited by Ian Chilvers
A Concise Oxford Dictionary of Mathematics
Christopher Clapham
The Oxford Spelling Dictionary   compiled by R. E. Allen
A Concise Dictionary of Law   edited by Elizabeth A. Martin

RECREATIONS IN MATHEMATICS

Recreations in Mathematics covers all aspects of this diverse, ancient, and popular subject. There are books on puzzles and games, original studies of particular topics, translations, and reprints of classical works. Offering new versions of old problems and old versions of problems thought to be new, the series will interest lovers of mathematics—students and teachers, amateurs and professionals, young and old.

THE PUZZLING WORLD OF POLYHEDRAL DISSECTIONS

Stewart T. Coffin

This fascinating and fully illustrated book examines the history, geometry, and practical construction of three-dimensional puzzles. Containing solid puzzles, such as burrs, Tangrams, polyominoes, and those using rhombic dodecahedron and truncated octahedron, this collection includes a variety of unsolved and previously unpublished problems.

MATHEMATICAL BYWAYS IN AYLING, BEELING, AND CEILING

Hugh ApSimon

Set in the fictional villages of Ayling, Beeling, and Ceiling, and requiring little formal mathematical experience, this entertaining collection of problems develop a wide range of problem-solving techniques, which can then be used to tackle the more complex extensions to each puzzle.

Also available:

The Mathematics of Games   John D. Beasley
The Ins and Outs of Peg Solitaire   John D. Beasley